The W

The weight management program used successfully by a group of California physicians since 1973

© 1990 by
Physicians Weight Management
6693 Folsom-Auburn Road, Suite E,
Folsom, California, 95630
Telephone: 916-988-5729
Email: www.weigh-out.com

ISBN 1-58909-154-X
Printed in the United States of America

Acknowledgments

Based on a concept by : A.T.Simeon, M.D. (Rome, Italy)

Medical Consultants: Elvira Lao, M.D.
Thomas Flectcher, M.D.
Grant Nugent, M.D.
Ron Stone, M.D.

Editorial Consultant: Betty Ford, Founder & Program Director

Program Trainer Kathy Platz

Complied & Written by: Sandra Parent

Edited by: Carmel Rooney

Cover Design: Parallax Design Group

Published by
eBookstand Books
Division of CyberRead.com
1687_6

TABLE OF CONTENTS

FOREWORD

This book was written to help you manage your weight at a safe and satisfying rate, and to help you maintain your "natural" weight —to give you new skills and working principles for a lifetime of habits you can live with comfortably.

This program is extremely effective, but it requires of you more than an initial impulse. No one has ever reached a goal, built a sailboat, closed a sale, or raised children merely on willpower or impulse. As with any priority in life, your desire, commitment, perseverance, and patience are required. Combine these with our proven successful program and you have the necessary skills to achieve your goal. Information is power. You can achieve anything you want with belief, commitment, and knowledge.

The care you give to understanding the principles outlined here and the conscientiousness with which you apply this knowledge to your personal weight management will determine how successful you are at losing your weight and keeping it off.

This book offers you an opportunity to regain control over your life. The degree of your success depends on your renewed choices and your renewed enthusiasm to begin for the last time!

The "right" diet for you can assist you not only in managing your weight but also in healing yourself, by helping you understand the issues that surround weight and the reasons that pounds accumulate in the first place. On the other hand, the "wrong" diet for you would be one that contributes to creating illness, failure, disappointment, avoidance, yo-yo-ing, undermining of you and your goals, and additional weight gain and leads to the sabotaging of your efforts once again.

No one diet program is the answer for everyone. Not only is everyone biochemically different, but each person has different needs and issues at different times.

If you have decided to lose weight, deal with the issues connected with it, heal yourself from the inside out, and make a commitment to do so, it doesn't matter what program or book you choose. Any of them could work. Once you have locked into and focused on your own path of what feels comfortable and right for you and your body, there is nothing that can stop you from making it happen.

DISCLAIMER

This book is designed to provide information in conjunction with the medically supervised weight loss program provided by this clinic. It is with this understanding that the information provided in this book is for your personal use only.

It is not the purpose of this book to reprint or duplicate any, or all, of the information that is otherwise available about weight loss, but to complement, amplify, and supplement the information provided by the physicians and medical staff here at the clinic. You are urged to read all the available material and learn as much as possible about weight loss, diets, nutrition, exercise, behavior modification issues, supplements, and any reputable subjects referring to the process of safe, effective weight loss.

Weight loss is not supposed to be a get-rich scheme, at your expense, but has been used to sell hundreds of lucrative programs and books for years, with no end in sight. This program has been used effectively for over twenty years by physicians and is not been available to the general public at this time. Many have expressed a desire to share this information with others. However, we would appreciate it if the information, with regards to this program, is not shared with others. This book is used in connection with the medical program and each person has individual needs and requirements.

Every effort has been made to make this book as complete and as accurate as possible. This text should be used only as a general guide and supplement and not as the ultimate source of weight loss and dieting information by or of itself. Furthermore, this book contains information on weight loss, nutrition, and related topics available only up to the printing date and until the next revision, at which time every effort will be made to provide even more current information on these subjects.

The purpose of this book is to educate, entertain, and inspire. The publisher shall have neither liability nor responsibility to any person or entity, with respect to any results or side effects caused, or alleged to be caused, directly or indirectly, by the information contained in this book, that is not used in conjunction with the medically supervised program. The decision to use this program, in conjunction or not, with other programs, with or without medical supervision, would be strictly at your own discretion.

DEDICATED TO:

THE SPIRIT WITHIN ALL OF US . . .

TO CHOOSE!

CHAPTER ONE

A New Way

2
BEFORE YOU BEGIN

The program begins with a visit to our medical office for a full physical examination and a consultation. At that time, our physician ascertains whether or not you qualify for the weight loss program. Oftentimes a person starts a weight loss program but is unaware that they may have undetected reasons that would delay or disqualify them to begin a diet. Education begins with a physician interpreting your lab work and your general health condition. Your proper nutrition, exercise, behavioral modification, and life style changes will be within the program book and discussed along with your specific program regimen.

Patients are comfortable on 1,000-1,200 calories per day with little or no hunger pangs or cravings. Women average 1/2 to 2 pounds a week weight loss, while men will average 2 to 4 pounds a week due to the differences in their hormones.

Weight loss is not just about "food"; Repeated dieting leads to greater difficulty in **losing** weight, greater efficiency in **gaining** weight and a tendency to overeat once food becomes available. One assumes that you don't have "conscious choices" about food while on a diet, or are being deprived of food **and** choices. This program addresses these "assumptions" on an ongoing basis.

Alot of patients (especially women) also start to retain water. After they discontinue a diet their bodies overcompensate and retain excessive water in and between the cells. With this "refeeding edema," as it is known, dieters suffer from chronic swelling. Moreover, the dieter often becomes confused and depressed in regards to continuing to make a commitment that ends up in failure. Despite adherence to a low-calorie diet plan, you can actually end up gaining weight instead of losing. Frequent dieting also lowers the metabolic rate (the number of calories you burn to support normal body functions).

Another aspect of the dieters' issues are that it may have become a way for some to "layer" or "protect" their sensitivities, feelings of pain, insecurity, old hurts, anger, self-worth, guilt, etc. The false sense of being able to "insulate" or "protect" along with "denial" and "resistance" can often keep weight on even with very little intake of food.

Variables like attitude, stress, climate, diet patterns, occupation, interpersonal relationships, chemical incompatibilities, commitment level, desire, motivation and the willingness to redesign lifestyles are all a part of "healing the whole person" from the inside out.

This program is also designed to distinguish between the different body fats. Only the abnormal fatty tissues are broken down as opposed to the lean muscle mass and the structural fat. This assures you that your body does not cannibalize its own tissue from starvation, which obviously would be self-defeating.

With all this taken into consideration, is it any wonder that at least one half or more of the adult population diets, and that 70% of those people will be "quick weight loss" repeaters? It's an epidemic of inappropriate dieting. People can't expect to alter their biology by starving. It's an epidemic of inappropriate dieting. People can't expect to alter their biology by starving in short or long periods of time. Any weight challenge, whether it's big or small, can do more than just affect your appearance. Your outlook and attitude on life are affected as well. Being overweight by as little as 10 to 20 pounds can often undermine a person's sense of confidence and self-worth.

In summary, we are concerned with treating the "whole" person. *Self-responsibility* is the focus. Education of your body's general condition and needs, nutrition, exercise levels, eating habits, negative beliefs and patterns, personal issues and self-support should be your focus. No longer should physicians just be held responsible for all the answers. Each person must take control of their choices about food and health on a daily basis, using physicians as only a foundation—not the mistakenly magic answer.

The purpose is to create an environment for you to begin your "last diet" and not be just another of the many statistics in the "repeat business" category. The commercial diet business has reached a $4 billion-a-year business—at your expense.

For over 26 years, this program has been instrumental in helping thousands of people achieve their goals, reach their *natural* weight, change life-styles, take back control of their lives, make *conscious choices*, accept responsibility for being the creator of their daily health and healings, and become a powerful representations to others, to support them in their decision to find a weigh out of the revolving diet door.

4

YOUR FOCUS SHOULD BE NOT ONLY TAKING THE WEIGHT OFF, BUT KEEPING IT OFF!

While that may seem a distant goal to you now, it is important to realize that this program is more than just a weight loss program. It is a four-part program designed to help you reach your goal and to maintain that goal for a lifetime.

The program has four phases:

1. Education
2. Weight loss program
3. Exercise
4. Maintenance

While each phase of the program is important to your success, this book has been prepared to assist and support you during our weight reduction program phase, which you are about to begin. However, all personal family physicians reserve the right to modify an individual's medical management in accordance with their own professional judgment.

Please remember that committed cooperation with the program, and with the advice or recommendations that our medical physician or staff may make, is very important to ensure your success.

'The way to win is to make it okay to lose.'

WHY THE PROGRAM WORKS

Always reviewing and updating the most current scientific and medically proven research and methodology on weight reduction and metabolism, our weight program has been modified to incorporate some of the past traditional methods along with newly discovered principles into a proven, safe, and highly effective program.

This is a four-part weight loss program:

1. **Education**—To begin, you learn to set realistic goals; understand your behavior with regard to your beliefs and habits about food; and foster a conscious awareness about making choices when eating, ordering, buying, and preparing food.

2. **Weight loss program**—The program centers around a low-calorie diet that has variety and is nutritionally well balanced. It is made up of a combination of foods that satisfy you to check, train, and re-educate your appetite. There are no calories or carbohydrates to count, and you will buy and prepare all of your own foods (from the foods allowed). Also you will be administered prescribed medications that will assist in appetite suppression, hunger control and support the lowering of your metabolism. (However, there are no amphetamines or controlled substances prescribed on this program.)

3. **Exercise**—Moderate, regular exercise is essential to losing weight. Exercise has been shown to increase the metabolic rate of fat calorie burning and to help reduce and lower the appetite. Not only does exercise work as a "handle" to crank down and stabilize your "set weight," but it will build lean muscle tissue and improve circulation and stamina. Exercise also reduces stress and tension and, in general, helps you to feel better and more fit. It's a habit that needs to become part of an everyday healthy life and is absolutely necessary for a healthy, consistent weight loss.

4. **Maintenance**—This step involves maintaining the acquired goal weight on an ongoing basis; support, information, and methods for ensuring permanent weight control; nutrition education, alternative eating options, and health guidelines; the nurturing process with special exercises; suggestions, recommendations, and knowledge regarding lifestyle health choices; and food for thought.

6

WHAT YOU CAN EXPECT
FROM THIS PROGRAM

1. Safe and consistent weight reduction averaging 1 to 2 pounds per week for women and 2 to 3 pounds per week for men

2. Little to no hunger after the first 2 to 3 days

3. High energy levels

4. A sense of well-being

5. Confidence that you are using a proven and safe method

6. Improvement or elimination of health risk factors associated with obesity, including high blood pressure, diabetes, fluid retention, arthritis, and elevated cholesterol

7. No calorie counting or complicated meal planning

8. Considerably lower costs compared to commercial weight reduction programs

9. Knowledge and learning skills that will remain with you for a lifetime

10. Support alternatives and education to resolve the conflicts and issues that accompany weight loss

11. Long-term management to maintain a "natural" weight

12. A new or renewed sense of being in control of your body, mind, and spirit

13. A guideline to making conscious choices

"Excuses are the lack of faith in your own power."

FAT IS NOT JUST ABOUT FOOD

It's about you challenging yourself.
It's about making conscious choices on a daily basis.
It's about fears and needs.
It's about who you are and where you want to be.
It's about the willingness to do what you have to do
to have what you want.
It's about honoring yourself.
It's about trusting your inner sense of knowledge.
It's about nurturing yourself.
It's about taking responsibility
for creating every moment of your life.
It's about living a life full of "wholeness."
It's about healing for the mind, body, and spirit
—from the inside.
It's about moving into a loving, supportive, nurturing,
growing, healthy lifestyle that you can call your own.
It's about a life that you will take full responsibility
for creating—or not creating.
It's about deciding that "there must be a better way."
It's about not being a victim anymore.
It's about avoiding—and not avoiding.
It's about finding "the way out."

Sandra

*"Each of us draws our own special circumstances to
ourselves, to provide unlimited opportunities
to learn, grow and fulfill our highest potential."*

*"Life was never meant
to be a struggle.
Just a gentle progression
from one point to another,
much like walking through
a valley on a sunny day."*

— Stuart Wilde

CHAPTER TWO

The Way Out

NEW ATTITUDES, NEW ALTERNATIVES

It is important to begin assessing some of the reasons, issues, and behaviors that are associated with your weight losses and gains. As you observe and become more aware of your emotional areas of uncomfortableness during this program, you will have an opportunity to re-evaluate your belief systems and life choices and perhaps make new decisions and better choices about changing and controlling them.

In this way, when you reach the maintenance portion of the program, you will be aware of the possible challenges and old habits that will rise to meet you once again when you have reached your "natural" weight. You will either choose to avoid and not change them or choose a new and more positive path.

We would like to see you confirm your commitments and goals and make new and positive decisions, new choices and habits, particularly in creating a new, positive, and powerful self-image. You also have the ability to nurture yourself and your lifestyle, to be patient and gentle with yourself, and to maintain a confident and secure feeling that you are in control of your life and your choices about your health and well-being.

As part of your commitment to your success and to set your "destination" or goal, take the time to complete the forms throughout the book to support yourself in establishing and maintaining realistic goals.

The decision to go beyond the physical and physiological areas of weight loss takes a special and determined commitment. Emotional issues that surround the gain and loss of weight can be very powerful. However, this particular program is not equipped with all the necessary tools and special skills to address many of these challenging and sensitive areas.

If you have a further interest in any of these subjects and would like to pursue a particular subject, many recommended books, tapes, and seminars are excellent sources for exploration in these areas. You can also find support groups and professionals in many fields in the yellow pages of your local phone book.

Commitment:

Commitment creates personal power.

Personal power creates choice.

Choice creates consciousness.

Consciousness creates awareness.

Awareness creates truth.

Truth creates freedom.

Freedom creates being.

Being creates you.

You create . . .

You!

Sandra

12

DEFINITION OF COMMITMENT

*'A promise or vow to do what you say you are going to do,
and to do whatever it takes to make that happen.'*

Making a commitment enables you to:

1. Prioritize your life

2. Focus your energy

3. Utilize your abilities and talents

4. Release your inner sense of power

5. Concentrate your skills and knowledge

6. Actualize your potential

7. Redefine your needs

8. Clarify your integrity level

9. Create your foundation of trust

10. Manifest your thoughts

11. Make conscious choices

12. See every crisis as an opportunity

13. Use criticism as a tool

14. Detach from external data

15. Self-contain your energy force

16. Direct your creativity

17.   Know your truths

18.   Understand accountability

19.   Create more commitments

20.   Be responsible for creating every moment of your life

21.   Accept who you are, where you are, and what you are

22.   Be aware of all your possibilities

23.   Challenge your limitations

24.   Move through restrictions

25.   Resolve conflicts

26.   Control your environment

27.   Recognize your issues

28.   "Create" your own life

"Commitment is what transforms a promise into reality. It is words that speak louder than words. It is making the time when there is none. Coming through time after time, year after year."

—*Shearson/Lehman*

14

"WHY DO I WANT TO REACH
MY NATURAL WEIGHT?"

Before writing these reasons down, give them some thought. It is important that they be very personal goals and desires. They should not be generalizations. They should be what you feel, not what you think would please others. These are used as guidelines in your program.

Take a few moments each day to read through your list. Revise it and redefine it as you become even more clear about the end results of your weight loss image.

Read the entire list whenever you are challenged with a difficult food situation. Reading the list reinforces your personal commitment to take control of your health and self-esteem.

1. _I'm tired of not feeling well_

2. _So I can be more comfortable with my body_

3. _____

4. _____

5. _____

6. _____

'There is no right or wrong, good or bad
—just different.'

GOALS AND COMMITMENTS

Name: _____Nancy_____ Date: _3/___

I will commit to: _stay with this program_

_____

first level

to reach the ~~natural~~ weight of: _170_ ~~by:~~ *in* _20 weeks_

(Please be realistic about your expectations)

My <u>natural</u> and permanent maintenance <u>weight</u> is: _140_

That may not realistic at my age.

When I reach my desired weight, I will not allow my weight to go

over _10 lbs_____, and if I do, I will correct it within _____

days.

When I reach _190_____ lbs., I will reward myself with:

a day at the Spa

_____

Signed: _Nancy_____ Date: _____

Commitment level: ___9.5____

(A level of 10 would be considered 100% committed!)

'To break bad habits,
you must acknowledge that you have them.'

16

LESLIE

I received a call from the program director of a local television station. He told me that his assistant, Leslie, was a bright, creative, and dedicated woman who had tremendous potential in television administration. There was just one problem. She weighed over 250 pounds. The additional weight contributed to her difficulty in breathing. Her frequent use of sick days because of ill health, and her low energy level. He needed someone who could keep up with him and with the demands of the job. He sincerely wanted her to get the help she needed to work toward her highest potential. He asked me if I would talk with her to see if the clinic could help her. I told him that I would be happy to try but that the only way she could be successful was if she were ready to take the responsibility of making the full commitment to lose that much weight.

Leslie came to the clinic the next morning. As we talked, I sensed that she was extremely uncomfortable, so I switched the topic of conversation to her job. She immediately became enthusiastic, and it was obvious that she felt her health and appearance were real threats to her position. When I asked her if she knew the reason why her weight seemed to be out of control her eyes filled with tears, and she told me that she really didn't know but that she did know that she had to do something. Her career was obviously the most important thing in her life. Her fears of failure added to her overall need to continue gaining weight to protect herself from the impending rejection. We agreed that she would take one day at a time and that the ultimate goal was to lose 100 pounds by the next Christmas in eleven months.

I kept track of her progress, but I didn't see her often because she came into the clinic very early. In September, I went to lunch with the clinic nurse. Right after we were seated, a charming woman stopped at our table to say hello. I didn't know that it was Leslie until she began to talk and I recognized her voice. She was an entirely different person. She exuded self-confidence, was beautifully groomed, and had a poised and assured presence about herself. This was not the Leslie I remembered meeting in my office. She told me that she had just returned from a national Broadcasters Association convention where she had represented her station as the new program director. Her former boss was now the station manager and obviously all of his support and faith had been rewarded. Leslie still visits us at the clinic now and then. She has had no problem maintaining her weight because she is in control now. She has sent many of her friends and colleagues to us, and they all continue to support each other and share their stories of success about not only about their weight, but about their lives.

CHAPTER THREE

The Way In

TO RISK

To risk laughing
is to risk appearing carefree

To risk weeping
is to risk appearing weak and childlike

To risk unfoldment
is to expose your vulnerability

To risk knowing yourself
is to risk knowing the truth

To risk committing to your ideas and dreams
is to risk actualizing them

To risk loving yourself
is to risk becoming whole and complete

To risk being still and listening
is to risk hearing what you need to do

To risk letting go
is to risk getting what you really want

To risk changing your life
is to risk living in the light

To risk going within
is to risk finding 'the way out.'

—Sandra

RISK

Any degree of risk has some element of the unknown, but no one courts risk without believing there is some chance to achieve what he or she sets out to do.

We sense when we are no longer able to ignore some inner voice: a feeling that prompts us to make the effort to begin to learn again, to change our lives, and to love ourselves.

Any risk, large or small, is intensely personal. It means decisions and personal challenges. Only we alone know, in the privacy of our hearts, what personal crisis we have conquered, or failed to; how big the mountain was that we attempted to climb, or climbed; and how long was the reach into the unknown.

The results of risks are commonly evaluated in terms of success or failure. But the true and valuable measure of risk is in what we have learned and how we have grown.

Once you have made a decision to risk at anything, the path will unfold before you, and the answers will move through you, from your heart, like a soft summer wind. Risking is being fully alive.

On the next page, make a list of what you are willing to risk and what you are not willing to risk to have what you want (weight loss, different job, new relationship, and so on).

'A friend lets you have your own truth.'

What are you willing to risk?

Trying again - again

Why? *Hope*

What else are you willing to risk?

Egg on my face - again

Why? *Hope*

What aren't you willing to risk? *Doing something stupid to loose weight*

Why? *my poor body deserves better*

What's the best that could happen if you were willing to risk?

I could succed

What's the worst that could happen if you risked?

I could fail — again

Are you willing to have things stay the same? *no*

Why or why not? *I'm sooo unhappy with me*

What could you learn form risking? *That I can succeed - finally*

What feelings come up when you consider risking? *fear - Hope - anxiety*

What is your personal truth about risking?

CHOICES

Often, because you assume that you don't have choices about food while on a diet, or after your diet program, some of you will eat just to satisfy the need to feel in control or to prove that you can't be told what to do.

Deprivation and restriction are big conflicts and issues for many of you on or off diets. When you start feeling restriction (as in choices of food) is when you will be most critical—of your diet, of yourself, or of those around you.

/ a demon, not friend !

Letting go of weight (pounds) will often be accompanied by the feeling of loss—the sense of losing a friend or a familiar supportive mechanism. Sadness is often part of this, as when you lose something or someone that has been a part of your life. Whether you are aware of it or not and whether it is a negative or positive influence, you may feel a sense of loss.

Being overweight may not have been what you wanted on a conscious level, but it was safe and was within your comfort zone. Even if the weight didn't feel good physically, it still served you in some way or may have been part of the need for protection or insulation from something or someone.

Often when we look back on seeming negative circumstances or unsupportive habits, the tendency is to condemn them. We find ways to be critical and try to erase or discard the residue of the experience from our memory.

Instead of dismissing it as a bad dream or incident, we should perhaps embrace this part of ourselves and our past. In discarding and discrediting it, we lose the ability to see the true value of its integrity in our life.

For instance, if it had not been for that particular person, situation, job, fear, habit, parent, spouse, health, challenge, or whatever the situation might be, you would obviously not have had the circumstances or the experience itself. Right? So without having the particular experience that environment provided, how would you have moved through the restrictions and limitations to reach the place where you are now?

Could it be that a particular time in your life actually did serve you and your growth? Even a time of unusual overweight?

As with a weight problem, when you lose the weight, you have a valid opportunity to look back and acknowledge how far you have come. Acknowledge that each pound you put on, as well as each pound you took off, served to validate the way you were and to bring you to where you are. Eventually, those pounds led you to the awareness that "this doesn't work for me," or "something is wrong with this picture," and "there has got to be a better way. . . this just isn't the way I want to be or the way I want my life to look."

Without each experience, you would still be stuck! Each experience brings you closer to who you really are—who you really want to be.

Forgive yourself and bless the pounds . . . each and every one. They served you well. Let go of the experience. Just don't forget that they were part of who you were and that human evolutionary experience allowed you to become who you are now!

Part of life is to experience restrictions and limitations. By going beyond those restrictions and limitations you come into your own personal power and freedom. Losing weight is choosing to step beyond whatever circumstances are connected to it.

Whatever you find difficult or arduous is almost always your main challenge at that time. It is the aspect that you have to go through to complete your experience with it. That is why adversity is so useful and powerful.

Think of all the times when you thought you wouldn't make it through a certain situation: losing weight, changing jobs, moving to another town, and so on. Then look at the growth and the wisdom that those times gave you. You could never have the knowledge and the awareness about yourself, your commitment level, or your inner strength that you have now, had it not been for those days of doubt and darkness. Those experiences were part of each path that you chose—and each path has led you to where you are today.

"You are really the only teacher you have ever known . . .
or will ever need to know."

ANSWERS

A wonderful by-product of any weight loss effort is the ability, in any situation, to stop and ask yourself: What is the truth about this? When an issue about eating, cheating, binges, anger, quitting, and the like occurs, you always have the option to make a choice!

There are only two rules to follow:

1. You must really want to know the truth.

2. Knowing the truth, you must make choices consciously.

Are you willing to know what choices you have and what the consequences are for making them—or not making them?

First of all, know that the answer, your personal truth, is always for your highest good and serves *your* intention to feel better about yourself.

But how do you know whether it's your ego or your inner self that is talking? It's very simple, and yet it is also something that takes time. It is simple because all you have to do is to listen. Listen to what your inner self is saying to you about any question that you ask.

The challenging part is to learn to discern the difference between your head talking and your heart feeling. It takes practice . . . but most of all, it takes trust.

Ask your question. Acknowledge that you really want to know the answer, and then just be still a moment. Usually the first impression you get will be your truth, your answer. Don't start analyzing it and don't try to figure out what it means. Just *be* with it a few moments.

If you want to try this, a fun way to begin and practice is with a simple trip to the grocery store. Pick up a particular produce or food item and hold it in your hand. Just feel it for a moment and then move the energy out of your head (thinking about it) and down into your heart area. Ask your body how it "feels" about this particular food item. Does it like it, or is it something that it doesn't need and or doesn't want? Then just listen. Usually the first answer you get is the truth about what you have asked. Pick up another item. Try it again. Then pick up two items, one in each hand, and feel which of the two is more compatible for you and your body.

Remember that you have to release and detach from the answer. If you have a vested interest or solid opinion about a particular food, you will probably have a more difficult time with the outcome of your answer. As an example, take a huge chocolate cake: You love the cake, but does your body like the cake? What is the price that both of you pay when you choose to have what won't honor you? Perhaps chocolate cake could be eaten in moderation if it is something that you can't live without. But choose to eat it consciously knowing that you do have other options.

Ask the question, release the need to be right or wrong, be willing to acknowledge the answer, and then just be still and listen. Be open and receptive, and, above all else, trust yourself and your body. You really do know what is for your highest good and in your best interest.

This little exercise can be used not only for food, but also for anything that you make choices about. You actually make choices every minute of the day about something. You are probably not even aware that you have not questioned many of your daily choices in the past and present.

Some simple examples of everyday choices are:
- lifting something that you know is too heavy for you;
- telling someone that you will help them out when you really had something else planned;
- saying yes to someone's invitation when you would rather be home with a good book;
- choosing a banana split instead of a fruit salad;
- buying something that someone else thinks is best for you, instead of making your own choice based on your own particular needs and desires;
- giving in to demands of the day when you just don't have any more to give;
- not allowing someone to help you, for fear that there is a price tag attached;
- telling someone what you think they should do instead of just listening to them;
- making judgments about something you've done instead of understanding that you've just learned something, forgiving yourself, and going forward.

No one knows what the truth is for you. But you must be willing to take responsibility for making or not making conscious choices with regard to your life. You really do know the truth.

You also know that there have been many times when you *did* know the truth but chose to suppress it. Did your choice honor you and who you really want to be? Or did it only make you resentful, guilty, or angry in the end?

The most difficult part of this exercise is the first step. The first time you ask yourself, recognize that there are many, many times when we already know the truth but unconsciously choose not to acknowledge it.

It's very possible that pounds are linked into this process. That is one of the reasons why your intentions are so important when you ask your questions. You must really want to know, and you should have a willingness to hear the truth. Even if you disagree with the answer or find a way to justify another answer, acknowledge that you do know the truth about what you have asked.

The answer may not make any sense to you in the beginning, but stay with it for a few moments before you discard it entirely. Most often, the very first words or whisper, or perhaps just a strong feeling, can give you tremendous insight about yourself and your question. The answer may come sometime during the day. It may be a sign that you look up and notice, and you just *know* that is your answer. It may be in a song on the radio, something someone says to you, or a line in a book. It can come from anyone, anywhere and any time. But you will know, on a deep, profound level, that it is the answer to what you asked.

Also, don't make judgments, opinions, or decisions about the answer. Keep your emotions detached. Treat it with a sense of interest, not with criticism. For this or any other process to work, you must try to understand, be compassionate, and above all, have patience with yourself and your ability to listen and hear.

Truth can only be experienced. It cannot be described or explained. Truth will dawn upon you in your own time. There is no more powerful teacher than your own truths! Your answers are just a whisper away.

At what point in your life will you make the statement
'there's got to be a better way'
—and then actually try to find it?

CHANGE

The natural state of being comes from inside and then expresses itself on the outside. As you come into a full, loving, and permanent acceptance of yourself from within, your body will have been gradually changing also. As fast as your inner self can accept that change, your body will not be far behind.

Any diet that you choose will eventually lead you into some type of change. Any process of weight loss means change.

For some of you, this will set up fears just in making the decision, just to know that whatever is going to happen will lead at some point into an area that will be different from what you know now.

For most of you, many things will change. For a few of you everything will change. In the beginning, you will need to acknowledge, or at least try to perceive, some sense of the changes in attitude, beliefs, programming, lifestyle, and environment that you think or believe will change for you in this weight loss process.

Many will never proceed from this point. The fear of change may be so great and so dominant in your life that the decision to change will be too fearful to make. Embarking on this decision could mean:

- not knowing what is going to happen,
- not being able to control the future,
- a new environment that might control your life, or
- moving into an unknown lifestyle.

To stay in control you must keep things the way they are, and to keep things the way they are . . . things cannot change. So you deny the fact that anything has to change.

Change creates the opportunities for growth and learning. Without change we become stagnant. The growth process is halted temporarily and we shut down to the possibilities that pass before us. Many are so afraid to change that they will actually choose an unhealthy state of being for their body and a dormant, lifeless existence over any changes. They choose to stay within the restrictions and limitations that they have control over, instead of incurring the unknown consequences of a change.

These particular people have had a long time to gather data and strengthen their position: They believe that they are right! One of the few ways that they are moved to change their minds is by way of a dramatic experience. They will be suddenly propelled into a crisis. During this experience, often they are given the opportunity to discover that they are not here to keep things the way they are but to awaken to their potentials and possibilities. The stress from a crisis provides the catalyst for a change to happen. The crisis could be a car accident, a disease of the body, a divorce, a job change, the death of a loved one, or many other possible events. When this occurs, the changing process could become the highest priority in these people's life.

Fear of success, control, and sudden changes are often involved with recognizing the inability to make changes easily.

However, for those of you for whom changing direction or shifting gears comes with ease, you most often will stop and start a diet process many, many times before you finally lock into a solid commitment to follow through and complete what you have started.

Follow-through and *completion,* for those of you that recognize your selves in this particular pattern, are the key words here. You will seldom finish or complete any project for one reason or another. Watch yourself in this scenario and see how many excuses you can come up with that justify not completing what you have started.

You will begin to see the same patterns with your diet commitment. Keep in mind that this is linked up with a restlessness in your process of thinking. You can change your focus of attention easily. When you are restricted from variety and change, you tend to become rebellious, and it is at these times that you will break with your project or commitment. Intimacy, confinement, and fear of restriction can often be linked to these areas.

Change is an important part of life. Being able to keep your commitments to yourself will probably mean some type of change. The need for a change may appear to come from an external source; however, your internal self in some way contributed to the necessity for some type of adjustment or adaptability to your new situation or commitment.

Some effort should be made to understand how you react to change, so that you can comprehend how changes in your body will trigger fear automatically.

Fear can accommodate and validate not wanting to keep your commitment by assisting you in becoming physically ill, creating a new crisis, or adding to your existing emotional stress.

When your body is threatened with change, it goes into a survival mode to uphold the old programming—the status quo. Recognizing this possible resistance could add to your awareness and strengthen your ability to stay committed. That's why it's so important to establish a solid commitment in the very beginning.

Before your body can begin to integrate new changes, mentally and physically, you may need to be prepared for the challenges your *body* could present to you—ways it also participates in the sabotaging of your efforts. Observe yourself; watch to see how you, your body, and your mind might be resisting.

Implementing changes happen in several phases. Here are some examples of the stages you may go through:

1.   Acknowledgment / Recognition of the need to change

2.   Denial that change is needed:

> There is nothing wrong with . . . .
> I can't do anything about this
> Nothing ever works
> It's hereditary
> I've been all right till now / I feel fine
> Even if I changed, life would still be the same
> Nobody cares what I look like anyway
> He/she loves me just the way I am
> I'm perfectly happy the way I am

3.   Resistance / Questioning the need / More resistance

4.   Disruption / Confusion

5.   Acknowledgment that there *may* be a need for change

6.   Surrender to the need-for-change issue

7.   Impatience—I want to have it change now!

8.   Adaptation—What will it feel like?

9.   What will I lose? What will I have to let go of?

10.   Survival—Will I die? Will I survive this change?

11.   Acceptance / Surrender to process (intermittent habit shift)

12.   Internalization of the change itself

13.   Shutdown—a time of rest and restlessness

14.   The shift takes place on a deep internal level

15.   Change is established, internally and externally

16.   Established routine of change becomes almost automatic

17.   Conscious acceptance of change in the daily habits

"Change is a prerequisite for growth."

"Dark is what grants light its existence, so don't ignore the dark.

"Dark is what grants light its existence, so don't ignore the dark.

You don't say that evil is bad, but rather that it highlights good or that it assists in creating goodness.

It's by dealing with who you are, who you have been, and what you have created in front of you that you go past the need to experience the challenge of negativity.

Once you totally accept that you, not fate, control your life, make your choices, consciously or unconsciously, a door opens silently within you and, without realizing it at first, you begin a higher evolution to freedom.

Your loss becomes your highest gain. Look at the present moment for your truth and allow the letting go of your old lies.

Release the past . . . let it go gently with the wind.

Become present in the now . . . in the moment with yourself . . . your true self.

There never really is any loss. We all are everything we ever were or are going to be when we are here in the now."

—Stuart Wilde

RESISTANCE

Have you ever postponed or procrastinated to any of these themes?

I'm not ready yet
I might fail
My friends would make fun of me
My spouse won't let me
I've already tried, and it didn't work
I may have to make changes
It costs too much money
Maybe after the wedding, divorce, etc.
I'm afraid to express my feelings
I don't want to talk about it
I don't have the energy
It's too limiting
It's just too hard to do
It's restricting
I still wouldn't be perfect
I don't have a doctor
I'm not good enough

Other forms of resistance may be seen in:

Changing the subject
Leaving the room
Going to the bathroom
Being late
Getting sick
Procrastination: doing something else
Doing busy work, wasting time
Looking away, or gazing out a window
Flipping through a magazine
Eating, drinking, smoking, etc.
Creating or ending relationships
Have breakdowns: cars, appliances, plumbing, etc.
I'll do it later
I can't think right now
I don't have the time right now
It would take too much time away from work, my husband, etc.
It's a good idea, but I'll do it some other time

I have too many other things to do
I'll start it tomorrow, next week, Monday, New Year's Day, etc.
As soon as I get through with . . . . I will . . . .
As soon as I get back from this trip, vacation, etc.
The time isn't right
It's too late, too soon, too early, etc.

And on and on the list goes. Do you recognize some of these as the ways you resist? *Look for the resistance in your excuses.*

Often, instead of working on our own changes, we decide which of our friends needs to change. This too is resistance. When something works well for us we often want to share it with others. But they may not be ready to make a change at that time.

It's hard enough to make changes when we want to, and even more difficult to try to make someone else change when he or she doesn't want to. This gets into the area of infringement. Stay focused on your own changes and allow others to make their choices about their changes in their own time. Instead of telling them what to do, represent what they *could* do.

If you are hesitant, resistant, or just don't want to change, ask yourself why. Don't scold yourself and don't find ways to punish yourself for not changing before. Just look at what you do and look for ways to begin doing it differently.

Be kind to yourself. Begin to love and approve of yourself and give yourself the time and the room to expand and change. Change does not come overnight. It comes with the willingness to have your life be different.

Remember, you are no longer helpless, you are not a victim. You are beginning a lifestyle of acknowledging your own power. You are starting to consciously make choices about how you want your life to look. If change in some way is part of that process, then take one day at a time and begin to make the changes.

There may be external effects to consider also. The effect of your making a change could affect those around you when you begin to make the changes. As you begin to change, it can often create fears for them. The interactions and impact on these individuals is crucial for you to be aware of and understand. They may try to sabotage your efforts just to keep the necessity for change out of *their* space— to keep their environment in the status quo.

34

A good communication process before you make your commitment will allow others to better understand and support you and your decision.

Instead of allowing them to sabotage your efforts, you need to ask family, friends, co-workers, and significant others for their support and understanding. Enlist them to help you in any way that they can. Assist them in their need for clarification. Tell them what your intention is and find out if they will be there for you.

'Truth cannot deal with lies that you want.'

LETTING GO

Part of the maintenance program is to let the past go as well as the pounds. The old image of yourself is replaced with the image you have chosen for yourself and your new lifestyle. Retain only the essence of what you have learned as you would remember the words of an old friend.

When you are frustrated with old thoughts and negative thinking, try to find a word or place that you can instantly relate to or draw on to replace it with. Focus on it until you are comfortable and feel in control again.

Still your thoughts for just a moment so that you can summon this feeling. Breathe deeply, relax, and let go of the fearful feelings. Find a way to dissipate them and dissolve their power over you once and for all.

Scales and charts are not necessary to know when you and your body feel comfortable. Most of you will come into an awareness of what feels "natural" as you get closer and closer to your goal weight.

Many of you are programmed into thinking that you have to set exact and perfect weight goals and have that "perfect" body in mind when you start. As you get closer to your true self, you'll begin to sense not only your "natural" body weight, but also a "naturalness" about who you are and everything you do.

You are actually in a series of gentle progressions of letting go. Many of the old weight beliefs and patterns and the many limitations and restrictions (most of which you were never even conscious of making a choice about) will begin to fall away as you drop your weight and move into a time of maintaining.

BEVERLY

Beverly's mother died a few months before she came to the clinic. She was still grieving and weighted thirty pounds more than she did at the time of her mother's death. Shortly after she started her program, I had an opportunity to talk with her. She was very sweet, in her late thirties, and had an excellent job with the state. She told me that she had never married because she believed it was necessary for her to take care of her mother. Listening to her speak of the demands that the mother had imposed on her and the mother's obvious alcoholism, I could see that she had been in an unhealthy, co-dependent relationship with her mother. Even with the death of her mother, she continued to play out the scenario. She would take care of relatives, friends, and co-workers, whoever she could find who "needed" help. As long as she had to keep helping someone else, she could continue to avoid helping herself. As she searched for yet another person to "need" her, her weight climbed to 260 pounds, and she realized that without help she would soon reach 300. She needed to find someone to help her.

As we continued to talk, she revealed a love-hate relationship with her mother. She was still overwhelmed with the grief and yet felt terribly guilty because she also felt a sense of relief. It seemed to be that the combination of guilt and need had to be resolved before she could really accomplish the task of losing weight. We talked every week, and she soon began to see that while her mother was in "need" of her care, Beverly herself also had a strong need to be needed. They both filled the need of the other. However, both needs were filled under negative and unhealthy conditions. In longing for someone to love, support, and care for her the way she did for her mother, Beverly contented herself with food as her mother had with alcohol. It was a closed and unconscious environment, with both addictions bringing each woman her own personal, but temporary comfort.

After Beverly was able to see the connection between her need for food and her need to feel needed by others, she was able to see the real need for a healthy, loving, and supportive relationship with herself. Coming to terms with the grief from the loss of her mother also gave her the awareness to face losing something else that was close to her—the fat. It was her insulation between her needs and someone else's. Beverly had to heal her self-esteem and be careful not to transfer her co-dependence for her mother to someone else.

Through time and patience, she began to put the pieces together that became the true picture of her whole self. She learned how to nurture herself, and to tend to her own needs. She lost 198 pounds, married a man she had worked with for years, and works on having interdependant relationships with her family and co-workers.

CO-DEPENDENCE

If you are one of the many individuals who grew up in a dysfunctional family, you no doubt have seen all the material and information available today with regard to co-dependence. Losing weight is a major issue that has been referred to as having a co-dependence connection. Co-dependents seem to share the same dynamics, behavior, and characteristics that result from growing up in wounding environments.

Many situations contribute to dysfunctional families. They run the gamut from violent chaos to rigid silence. Is it possible to identify some types of wounds that you may have received? Have you learned about family roles and the personality characteristics that result from childhood pain? Perhaps this is an area that you have related to and you have begun to find ways of healing that part of your life. You may also already be aware of how co-dependence and overweight may go hand in hand.

Becoming aware of family dynamics and learning to break the "don't talk," "don't feel," "don't trust" rules in a safe environment helps people validate their feelings and experiences. It can offer you new possibilities and help you make better choices about how you want to live. It can also contribute to healing the feelings of shame and disloyalty about revealing to others the truth about what happened; finding acceptance and understanding for yourself, and feeling less isolated and more like other people.

Dealing with co-dependence issues may have also helped you in seeing a clearer picture of the need to lose weight. More importantly, you will have taken a meaningful step toward connecting your co-dependent issues with weight, specifically your plateaus.

Growing up is not always easy, especially if you grew up in a family in which the communication skills of your parents were lacking or their expression of love was very conditional and controlling. These conditions create wounding, dysfunctional environments.

Co-dependence can be found in many forms. Relationships such as with parents, spouses, children, friends, and co-workers are only a few of the ways that we set ourselves up in co-dependent situations.

Co-dependence creates many opportunities for avoidance and excuses for weight gain. Being able to identify what holds you in these patterns may help you to discover what issues you are using your weight to protect you from. The connection remains one of externalizing life and its circumstances, which creates a vacuum inside and thus the need for insulating the emptiness, pain, guilt, and other feelings within.

A major fear could be that if you didn't have that connection and obligation to the other person(s), you would then become responsible for your own environment and personal experiences. This is where the inadequacy and feelings of "not being good enough" will seep into the outer realms of consciousness to move you back into dependency each time you attempt to pull away (each time you start a diet).

People who spend most of their time saving, nurturing, caring for, or being responsible for others in a co-dependent relationship have learned to shift their energies and time to those others instead of spending it on themselves.

Serving others because of guilt, programming, beliefs, and soon is another way to get the focus off your own issues and move the attention onto someone else.

If you really look at these particular types of situations, you may find that you "bought into" the situations for your own needs to be served . . . not the other person's. The ability to control someone through a guilt factor is very attractive. You may do what you need to do just to hold on to your position of control. Losing weight may mean you would lose control. Your focus, then, would be on yourself and not on controlling the situation.

And you may find out that you are not needed—that others really are capable of surviving without you. Or you might have to achieve or accomplish what you said you always wanted to do (if only you had the time and didn't have to take care of others in some way): write that book, go back to school, open a business, lose weight, travel, or whatever. Of course, when faced with the reality of actually doing it, you risk the possibility of failure.

Co-dependence is a crippling device for everyone involved. It serves as a wall to keep you from actualizing your full potential. It's a powerful tool to keep growth and change away from your door, and it provides you with still another opportunity to sit back and restrict and limit yourself from being all that you are meant to be.

If you have ever tried to break away from a co-dependent relationship, it's very possible that you will have recognized an abundance of resistance from those that you take care of or "save" on a regular basis.

Perhaps when you have tried in the past to reclaim your power, you found that you came face to face with feelings of not being needed, not being a good mother or father, not being the perfect spouse, not being a wonderful daughter or adequate son, not having any value, losing control, guilt, and so on.

But, more than likely, you managed to make yourself feel that you didn't deserve the time, attention, or nurturing that you were attempting to experience. You may have unconsciously found ways to either stay in the game or sabotage any efforts of others to pull out of the situation. Either way, both sides eventually become locked into stagnation and denial.

There are many advantages for holding onto co-dependent situations. Not having to find a way to fulfill your own needs is often one of the best. The beginning of healing for this particular issue, as with any issue, is to acknowledge that you are possibly in a co-dependent relationship, that in some way you are imposing your beliefs and needs on someone else, that in reality you have probably unknowingly set up a self-serving situation for the benefit of your needs.

Whether it be with family, friends, addictions, yourself, or even with your co-workers, it is necessary to recognize that somewhere in your past lies a scene that has become your method of operation or your "picture of life." You are the only one who that can change the way you want the picture to look now.

Look at the possibilities of why you have the same scenario repeated again and again in some way or another in your life. Don't make a judgment about it. This is not another reason to validate that you're not o.k. However, it could be another opportunity to change the way you think your life has to be. It is just part of the many masked opportunities that present themselves to allow you to experience the way that you give your power away to others. It also offers you the adventure of taking your power back.

This may be the place where you face why you gave up all the other times that you attempted to deal with your weight problem. Look at what comes up for you in this type of situation. Confront the fear of what would happen if you withdrew from a co-dependent relationship. Would you just find another way to set yourself up to serve someone or something else, or would you be willing to move into a recovery process and begin to heal the wounds?

Again, ask yourself if your lifestyle situation and relationships with yourself and others are serving you or serving an archaic need based on inadequate information and valueless motives. Do all your relationships honor and nurture you?

If you are in a co-dependent relationship, have acknowledged it, and are willing to heal the old wounds and reclaim control over your own life, you are on the path from fear to freedom.

Co-dependent books are listed in the "Suggested Reading" section at the back of the book.

'Every loving thought is true.
Everything else is an appeal for healing and help,
regardless of the form it takes.'

PROTECTION

Fat may have become your protection from anything you need to be protected from: men, women, sexuality (blossoming or developed), frightening feelings of any sort, emotional or physical abuse, childhood fears, relationships, intimacy, love . . . the list goes on.

Fat can often become your way of rebelling, your way of telling your parents, friends, lovers, significant others, the society around you that you don't have to be who they want you to be.

Fat can become your way of talking. It says: "I need help," "go away," "come closer," "I can't," "I won't," "I'm angry," "I'm sad," "I've been hurt, abused, not worthy, not lovable," and the personal universal favorite, "I'm not good enough." It may have become a vehicle for dealing with problems that you don't want to confront.

If you take away the fat without uncovering the needs it is expressing, you are left without a way to say what you do or don't want to, or don't know how to, or feel you can't say directly. Fat speaks for you. In our culture it may appear to be, or feel like, it is unacceptable to be fat, which makes it seem self-destructive to continue to be overweight.

Fat can feel like it is regarded as a deviation from the norm; it is sometimes regarded as or considered unhealthy or undesirable. Fat shows; it is unavoidable and apparent. And it is precisely because it is a deviation, because it sticks out, because it is so devastating to be fat in a thin society, that fat serves its function as communicator so well.

Eventually, you may feel so much guilt, the situation may get so painful, or your health may become so compromised that you become willing to listen to what the fat is saying to you instead of the real truth that will give you freedom.

Like carrying a baby around who just won't make its way down the birth canal, your fat, though uncomfortable, is familiar and safe. Is there something comforting about your discomfort—the familiarity of it? After a while, the solace of it will fade away. When the familiarity is not enough to keep you wrapped around yourself, you may begin to question whether your weight is still acceptable to you and whether it's just about food. Letting go of and finally releasing the all-too-familiar fat, like a baby, may bring on feelings of loss, a sadness that is not easily understood—the postpartum blues of weight loss.

THE PLATEAU

A Three-Step Process

LEVEL ONE: Acknowledging and identifying that a plateau exists

The plateau can represent the strongest point of holding on to an old pattern. Usually this is directly connected with the circumstances surrounding a previous time when you maintained a particular weight for a specific amount of time.

There are a multitude of reasons, emotionally as well as physically, that may be a part of any plateau: Money struggles, job crisis, relationship problems, stress are a few of these.

Many times such incidences as date rape, sexual assault, childhood molestation, physical or emotional abuse have never been dealt with and healed. The experience and feelings were shielded and protected by layer upon layer of fat that served as insulation for the wounds against the outside world.

Strong patterns of denial and justification may exist at this point to help you find excuses and reasons to go off your diet. It may seem too scary to bring such issues to the surface, along with the possibility that you may experience the pain and hurt that accompanied the original experience.

You may simply think you can't maintain the diet. Pain, hurt, anger, lack, resentment, and confusion are just a few of the feelings that may come up for you during this holding pattern at a certain weight without you being fully aware of them.

Actually, this is where the window awaits you. This is where you will be given the opportunity to push through the barrier and proceed into the next level. At this threshold is where you would most likely discontinue or quit your diet.

Most commonly, this can be the old pattern's and habits' strongest moments. Also, denial, excuses, justifications, guilt, and lack of a strong commitment lie within this time zone.

You will meet your particular level of commitment here. This is a time when you will have to go within to maintain a sense of being firmly committed and reaffirm that your intentions are clear. You must also decide whether to pursue avenues of support at this time. Only you know what you need to do to assist yourself to open the window or to lock it.

LEVEL TWO: Choosing to see through the window

Whether you choose to see through the window to the opportunity that lies on the other side of the plateau is the challenge. It is also the turning point for you and your commitment.

To give up and try it again at another time when you think that you might be stronger or when "it will just be a better time" —this is one of the of many dialogs or conversations you may hear from inside.

Often during this period you will allow your perseverance and nurturing to lag behind, with the result that you are not being supported and nurtured to keep you strong in your convictions.

The difficulty may be to maintain a sense of the end result: the sense of faith and trust that the block will eventually move and allow you to pass through the old fear or programming and into the next level of weight loss.

This may be a very delicate and difficult time for you. It will be very important to nurture and have patience with yourself. Recognize that this is a time of healing—healing your whole self, not just the physical, fat part of you.

It's important to have some type of consistency to remind yourself to stop in the moment and look back periodically. Take a look at where you are in your healing process from a higher perspective. Acknowledge again how far you have come, not how far you have to go.

Remember, this is not just a diet. It is a process of healing the whole person—not only your body but also your thoughts, habits, views of life, belief systems, and pictures of how you choose your life to be, not how you were told or how you perceived or programmed that it was suppose to be. This is also a time to acknowledge how far you have come and where you've made have a choice to be when you are finished.

Your goals and reasons will change as you get closer. The closer you get to where you want to be, the more you will find that the road you have traveled to get there has value, not just the end of the road.

Your concentration and focus at this time are also a major factor.

44

Concentration consists of two parts: consistency and density. Consistency is, basically, layering one thought form on top of another—just as you have layered your weight one period of time after another.

Consistency is coming up with something you want, holding that intention, and layering one new thought over the next and another over that. Gradually moving in a measured way with a measured step, layering one thought form upon another, at the same time removing one layer of fat at a time and then another, at each plateau. This allows a concentration of thought forms around us that holds the intention.

As the fat layers are one by one removed, they lose their power, control, and significance.

This is why the plateau can be so vitally important to your progress. Each one represents a new level, a new window that has been opened, and a renewed sense of power each time it is accomplished. Instead of materializing the old identity of yourself by the pounds on your body, you will begin to identify with your inner self. You will indeed begin to feel that a real power is within yourself.

Each time you pass through the window of the plateau you will be gaining the momentum of knowing that you will make it through the next one and the next one. You become stronger and more powerful in your intention and your commitment. You will recognize that you are creating your world. This knowledge and inner sense of self will carry you forward until you reach a point where you will actually welcome the plateaus in expectation of the next opening.

LEVEL THREE: Allowing your body to make an internal shift

You need to understand that at these times, perhaps, the consciousness finds it necessary to slow you down in some way, for a brief time to stop the input of information and begin a kind of "internal shift." This kind of shift moves your entire perception on the particular issue or fear that you are working with, into a new, different, and permanent position and perception, one that you have decided or chosen consciously. Maybe your consciousness just needs this time to assimilate and make the changes in your attitude, beliefs, programming, perception, patterns, and habits.

To do this, your mental, emotional, and physical body disconnects

45

from this reality in some way and goes within itself to redefine and reissue new data regarding the new choice: to heal itself from the inside out, then to surface and reconnect with your everyday reality.

When this process is finished, you might look back upon the past few moments, days, or weeks and see that you were walking around on automatic . . . in a fog, just going through the motions in a mist. At this point, you may feel a clearing . . . a crystallizing of your thought process and a renewed sense of your commitment. Your self-awareness and your personal power will be at their highest.

It is very important at this point that you really be with and acknowledge your feelings. You need to really feel them and remember them well. Remembering your feelings will serve as a focal point when you are at the threshold of yet another window.

'The most sacred road on earth
is where an ancient hate
has become the present path of love.'

SUZANNE

I heard the nurse ask Suzanne "Have you ever been at this same weight before?" That question, in our clinic carries with it the opportunity for a "breakthrough." As Suzanne was leaving, I asked her if she was able to recall any specific time in her life when she was at the same weight at any other time in her life. She told me that she couldn't remember and that she was on her lunch hour and had to get back to work. As she was leaving, she exclaimed, "I remember." She said it had just come to her in an overwhelming wave of emotion that she had weighted around 140 pounds when she was going through her divorce. With that, she turned and went back out the door. I informed the nurse, and when Suzanne came in the following week, she and the nurse discussed all the events surrounding Suzanne at the time of her divorce. She said that it had been very emotional and that she carried a lot of pain from the experience.

Suzanne had married her childhood sweetheart. Her husband had criticized and devalued her time spent on homework and volunteer time, consequently, she quit nursing school. Since the divorce, she has finished school, become a specialized pediatric nurse at a local hospital and gained an additional twenty pounds. One evening she was watching a movie called Irreconcilable Differences. In the movie before and after the divorce, the woman in the movie gained weight and became obese. Suzanne was stunned . She saw her own reflection on the TV screen as well as the one in the television movie. She too had used her eating as a way to numb the pain after the divorce. Each time Suzanne had a setback or someone criticized her or she started something new, the weight would begin to climb yet again. She realized that she had never admitted to herself that she had made the choice to quit school and that she took constructive criticism as personal rejection. It became especially difficult each time she started to lose weight. The old fears of starting something and not completing it, coupled with feelings of not being good enough, would come flooding back. Her fear of the pain and rejection would compel her to quit or sabotage any previous efforts to finish a weight program. After the discussion with the nurse, she began to lose weight again. She began to see the strong connection between the weight and the insulation from the old situation and the feelings tied to it. She wasn't going through a divorce; she had finished school and she had learned to handle constructive criticism from fellow students and teachers. Suzanne had several days of emotional upheaval and discomfort before she was able to convince herself and her body that she was in deed in charge and that everything was going to be all right. There was no need to protect herself from the "old movies" of her past. She released them along with the pounds and completed the program.

*The following pages are excerpted from
Louise Hay's book,* You Can Heal Your Life.

OVERWEIGHT

Overweight is another good example of how we can waste a lot of
energy trying to correct a problem that is not the real problem. People
often spend years and years fighting fat and are still overweight. They
blame all their problems on being overweight.

To me, overweight is a fear and a need for protection. When we feel
frightened or insecure or not good enough, many of us will put on
extra weight for protection. To spend our time berating ourselves for
being too heavy, to feel guilty about every bite of food we eat, to do
all the numbers we do on ourselves when we gain weight, is just a
waste of time. Twenty years later we can still be in the same situation
because we have not even begun to deal with the real problem. All
we have done is to make ourselves more frightened and insecure, and
then we need more weight for protection.

The diet that does work is a mental diet, dieting from negative
thoughts. I say to clients, "Let us just put that issue to one side for
the time being while we work on a few other things first." They will
often tell me they can't love themselves because they are so fat, or as
one girl put it, "too round at the edges." I explain that they are fat
because they don't love themselves.

When we begin to love and approve of ourselves, it's amazing how
weight just disappears from our bodies. Sometimes clients even get
angry with me as I explain how simple it is to change their lives. They
may feel I do not understand their problems. One woman became
very upset and said, "I came here to get help with my dissertation, not
to learn to love myself." To me it was so obvious that her main
problem was a lot of self-hatred, and this permeated every part of her
life, including writing her dissertation. She could not succeed at
anything as long as she felt so worthless. She couldn't hear me and
left in tears, coming back one year later with the same problem plus
a lot of others.

Some people are not ready; and this is not judgment of them. We all
begin to make our changes in the right time, space, and sequence for
us. I did not even begin to make my changes until I was in my forties.

So here is a client who just looked into the harmless little mirror, and
he or she is all upset. I smile with delight and say, "Good! Now we are

48

I talk more about loving the self, about how, for me, loving the self begins with never, ever criticizing ourselves for anything.

I watch their faces as I ask them if they criticize themselves. Their reactions tell me so much: "Well, of course I do. All the time." "Not as much as I used to." "Well, how am I going to change if I don't criticize myself? Doesn't everyone?" To the latter I answer, "We are not talking about everyone; we are talking about you. Why do you criticize yourself? What is wrong with you?" As they talk I make a list. What they say often coincides with their "should" list. They feel they are too tall, too short, too fat, too thin, too dumb, too old, too young, too ugly (the most beautiful or handsome will often say this), or they're too late, too early, too lazy, and on and on. Notice how it is almost always "too" something. Finally we get down to the bottom line and they say, "I am not good enough." Hurrah, hurrah! We have finally found the central issue.

They criticize themselves because they have learned to believe they are "not good enough." Clients are always amazed at how quickly we have gotten to this point. Now we do not have to bother with any of the side effects, such as like relationship problems, money problems, or lack of creative expressions. We can put all our energy into dissolving the cause of the whole thing: not loving the self.

Overweight represents a need for protection. We seek protection from hurts, slights, criticism, abuse, sexuality, and sexual advances; from a fear of life in general and also specifically. Take your choice. I am not a heavy person, yet I have learned over the years that when I am feeling insecure and not at ease, I will put on a few pounds. When the threat is gone, the excess weight goes away by itself.

Loving and approving of yourself, trusting in the process of life, and feeling safe because you know the power of your own mind make up the best diet I know of. Go on a diet from negative thoughts, and your weight will take care of itself.

Too many parents stuff food in a baby's mouth no matter what the problem is. These babies grow up to stand in front of an open refrigerator saying, "I don't know what I want," whenever there is a problem.

However, I would not blame our parents for this. We are all victims of victims, and they could not possibly have taught us anything they did not know. If your mother did not know how to love herself or your father did not know how to love himself, then it would be impossible for them to teach you to love yourself. They were doing the best they could with what they had been taught as children. If you want to understand your parents more, get them to talk about their own childhood; and if you listen with compassion, you will learn where their fears and rigid patterns come from. Those people who "did all that stuff to you" were just as frightened and scared as you are.

The following list of mental equivalents has been compiled from many years of study, my own work with clients, and my lectures and workshops. It is helpful as a quick reference guide to the probable mental patterns behind the disease in your body. I offer these with love and a desire to share this simple method of helping to heal your body.

We have listed only a few. The following are the most common areas for overweight. Look through the list and pinpoint the specific area where you hold the most weight. Then look at the mental description that Louise Hay feels is the mental equivalent. Often you will recognize a description that you can relate to your weight issue. If you would like to see the entire list (which also lists the "new thought pattern" for each problem) or have an interest in reading *You Can Heal Your Life*, it is listed at the back of this book.

PROBLEM	SUGGESTED EMOTIONAL COUNTERPART
CELLULITE	Stored anger and self-punishment
CHOLESTEROL	Clogging the channels of joy, fear of accepting joy
DEPRESSION	Anger you feel you have no right to have, hopelessness
DIABETES	Longing for what might have been, a great need to control, deep sorrow, no sweetness left
EDEMA	What or whom won't you let go of?

FAT (GENERAL)		Oversensitivity; often represents fear and shows a need for protection; fear may be a cover for hidden anger and a resistance to forgive
FAT	Arms	Anger at being denied love
	Belly	Anger at being denied nourishment
	Hips	Lumps of stubborn anger at the parents
	Thighs	Packed childhood anger, often rage at the father
HEART PROBLEMS		Long standing emotional problems, lack of joy, hardening of the heart, belief in strain and stress
HEARTBURN		Fear, fear, fear; clutching fear
HOLDING FLUIDS		What are you afraid of losing?
OVERWEIGHT		Fear, need for protection; running away from feelings; insecurity, self-rejection; seeking fulfillment

"Healing is on the other side of fear."

CECILIA

I met Cecilia at one of our satellite clinics on the first day she started the program. She came in faithfully for six months, but the nurse working with her was frustrated because Cecilia was making no progress. Her weight fluctuated only ten or twenty pounds of her starting weight every month. I made it a point to talk to her on several occasions, and she was polite but defensive when we discussed her lack of progress. Finally, I asked her if she would be willing to talk to Sandra to see if the two of them could find out what the difficulty was. She put it off for several weeks but finally consented.

Sandra discovered in their session an issue in Cecilia's childhood that she had never been willing to deal with. They got to the heart of the issue on that same day. Cecilia didn't come back for three weeks. When she did return, she came into my office and asked if she could restart her program and I assured her that we would be delighted to help her to try again. She began to lose weight that first week and continued to do so until she reached her goal. She lost ninety pounds and dropped nine dress sizes. She told me her friends didn't recognize her, and some of them had dropped her. She understood that they no longer felt comfortable around her because she now represented what they wanted to accomplish and become.

Cecilia learned to face her childhood trauma and understand that she was using her weight as protection to prevent the trauma from ever happening again. As long as she had her "fat" around her no one could get to her. The "fat" kept everyone at a distance, literally and figuratively. Once she began to work through the fear, she was able to put the shame and guilt behind her, place the responsibility on the people who owned it, and get on with the living of her life. She was no longer willing to have the past dictate her everyday decisions. She acknowledged that she was an adult who could say no, could protect herself, and would not allow anyone to get close to her again without her permission. She would never be a victim again.

Several months after she had finished her program, she was even able to confront the people who had instilled the fear that had controlled her life. Cecilia now helps others as a volunteer and has a understanding of what contributes to creating the weight issues in so many women. She also has a wonderful sense of peace about her now, and others love being around her. Her fear has been transformed into strength and deep compassion for others and their weight challenges.

"Waving good-bye,
leaving and smiling,
I release old energy.
I walk confidently into the new day."

- Stuart Wilde

CHAPTER FOUR

The Weigh In

GETTING STARTED

You must eat only the foods allowed on the program. The manner in which these calories, proteins, food groups, and carbohydrates are made up is thoroughly researched, proven, and very specific for your most effective weight loss results.

The diet is very closely balanced for you in calories, carbohydrates, fibers, and nutrition. Compromises or substitutions should not be made.

Because of the extreme sensitivity of the balance set up by this method, even a small amount of food not on the diet may cause a weight gain out of proportion. It may take days before it shows up and then 2-3 days to stabilize again. This may also trigger hunger and perhaps a feeling of lethargy. Before you let this happen, ask yourself if that extra bite or drink is worth the possible setback. The long-term gratification of the weight loss is much more lasting, positive, healthy, and encouraging than the short-term gratification of eating something off the diet.

The program will last only a short period and is a very small portion of time in your life. You are not restricted to certain foods forever, only for a short time, and the rewards, benefits, and satisfaction are long term and well worth the effort.

During the first few days of the diet, patients often tell us they feel better than ever and have extra energy, a sense of clear-headedness, and a feeling of "lightness." This general sense of well-being continues throughout the program.

If you strictly follow the specified diet and the recommended program regimen, you will find that not only is it easy and uncomplicated, but also extremely satisfying and even enjoyable.

"If you don't start—
it is certain that you won't arrive."

FATS

Three Kinds of Fat

To explain the cause of obesity, we will briefly outline the three kinds of fat so that you may better understand this basic concept of fat metabolism.

1. Structural Fat

Structural fat is like packing material; it fills the various gaps between the organs and acts like a bedding in protecting them. It is responsible for keeping the skin smooth and taut, and padding the bones and joints. This is a normal type of fat and is very undesirable to lose. A loss of this type of fat by intense dieting often results in joint pains, painful feet, and especially painful heels. Painful heels are often blamed on bone spurs but are actually the loss of normal fat pads under the heel bones. Nature intended the fat pad to be there to cushion the weight of the body.

2. Normal Reserve Fat

The normal reserve fat serves as an energy storehouse upon which the body may draw when intake is insufficient to meet demand. This is the so-called mobile fuel fat, readily available to supply energy when needed. These normal reserves are distributed throughout the entire body. This is a normal type of fat and is not desirable to lose, since it is needed for supplying energy in nutritional emergencies such as illness, nausea, vomiting, and so on.

Even if the body stocks both type 1 and type 2 fat to the maximum capacity, the individual still would not be called obese or even appear fat.

3. Brown's Adipose Tissue Fat (or Abnormal Accumulated Fat)

Type 3 fat occurs in the obese person. It also serves as a reserve fuel like type 2 fat, but unlike the normal reserve, it is not readily available to the body in nutritional crises. It is locked away in a fixed deposit and is not kept in a readily available "current account" like the normal reserve fat. It is deposited typically in areas such as the abdomen, hips, thighs, and upper arms.

THE LOADING DIET
BEGINNING THE PROGRAM
(This diet is to be used the first two days only!)

This part of the diet program is very important to your weight loss success. The loading diet is designed to supply your body with the proper amounts of the specific foods needed. This will also assist your system to begin to mobilize fats and to decrease excess water retained. It is high in protein and very low in carbohydrate but is extremely beneficial in getting your system and diet off to a great start. Please follow the instructions as carefully as possible for this two-day period. These two days will also give you an opportunity to read through your book and plan and prepare for the regular diet program that will begin on the third day.

THE LOADING DIET - THE FIRST TWO DAYS

1. Follow this loading diet for the first two days only.
2. It is very important you *do not* have any carbohydrates (i.e., fruits, breads, rice, potatoes, cereals, pasta, desserts etc.) unless your physician has instructed you otherwise.
3. Eat as much of the allowed foods, on the list, as you need *to satisfy your appetite.*
4. It is important that you are *not hungry* (but *do* quit eating when you are full).
5. Begin drinking the 2 quarts of water daily required on the program. If you are not used to drinking this much liquid, then work up to drinking 2 quarts (64 oz.). You might have 32 oz. the first day, 48 oz. the second day, and so on. **WATER IS ESSENTIAL TO THE SUCCESS OF THE PROGRAM.**
6. Any of the liquids, condiments, or seasonings listed in the diet section of the program book are okay to use on these two days of the loading diet.

IF AT ANY TIME DURING THE TWO-DAY PERIOD THE LOADING DIET DOES NOT AGREE WITH YOU, BEGIN THE REGULAR DIET PLAN IN THE PROGRAM BOOK.

First, read the entire book. The first two days you begin the program, read through the loading program itself again and become familiar with the regular diet plan. Take the time to complete the section on commitments and goals. Write down any thoughts that you may have during this beginning stage. They can be used later to encourage you during a time when you may not remember how determined you were in the beginning.

LOADING DIET—THE FIRST TWO DAYS

THE FOODS LISTED BELOW CAN BE EATEN IN ANY QUANTITY DESIRED UNLESS SPECIFIED OTHERWISE. DO NOT EAT ANY FOODS THAT ARE NOT ON THE LIST.

PROTEINS: All proteins may be broiled, barbecued, braised, or baked. Not fried, glazed, or cooked in gravy or sauce. Trim off excess fat or skin before cooking.

BEEF (ALL VERY LEAN): Steak (flank, porterhouse, filet mignon, sirloin, T-bone, rib roast, prime rib, roast beef, rump roast). No ribs or hamburger.

VEAL OR VENISON: Lean and trimmed of fat.

CHICKEN OR TURKEY: Light meat only (breast preferred). Remove skin before cooking and eating. Not fried, dipped, or coated. Lean ground is okay.

FISH AND SEAFOOD: Steamed or poached in addition to the above methods of cooking. Not dipped, coated, breaded, fried, with sauces or butter: Bass, butterfish, bluefish, cod, crab, flounder, grouper, haddock, halibut, kingfish, mahi mahi, octopus (squid or calamari), orange roughy, prawns, salmon, seabass, shad, shrimp, smelt, sole, sturgeon, swordfish, shark, trout, turbot, tuna, and whitefish. No abalone, oysters, clams, mussels, eel, fishsticks, sardines, or escargot (snails).

DUCK, PHEASANT, DOVE, QUAIL, OR SQUAB: Cooked as above. Remove skin.

EGGS: Any form (if fried or scrambled, use PAM or similar product—no butter). Limit egg use if your cholesterol is over 200.

VEGETABLES - 2 SERVINGS EACH DAY

1 SMALL SALAD WITH CHOICE OF NONFAT DRESSING
(Limit dressing to 3 tablespoons)

OR

2 CUPS OF STEAMED VEGETABLES
Only use vegetables from the list below:
Bean sprouts, broccoli, brussel sprouts, cauliflower, celery, cucumbers, lettuce (all varieties), mushrooms, onions, radishes, tomatoes, zucchini

HEALTHY SELF =

HEAL * THY SELF

CHAPTER FIVE

The Weigh Out

GENERAL INSTRUCTIONS

Read the diet instructions carefully. Reread them daily for the first week and frequently after that. Don't rely on your memory. The success of the program depends on how closely you follow and adhere to the diet and the rules.

THIS DIET SHOULD BE FOLLOWED
AS CLOSELY AS POSSIBLE!

1.   Make no substitutions or deviations.

2.   Foods eaten that are not on the diet may stimulate hunger or cause weight gain.

3.   Eat all the recommended foods from each of the food groups to ensure adequate nutrition, variety, and a feeling of well-being and energy.

4.   Record everything you eat and drink.

5.   Exercise a *minimum* of three days per week, 30 minutes per day.

6.   Take a multivitamin-mineral supplement daily.

7.   Limit the use of salt as much as possible.

8.   Alcoholic beverages are *not* allowed.

9.   It is imperative that you drink the required amount of water daily (2–3 quarts).

10.   Don't shop when you're hungry. Bring a list of the allowed foods with you if necessary.

11.   If you don't eat all the food portions for one day, you may not save the remaining portions for the next day.

12.   Notify the nurse of any change in your present medications, including over-the-counter, or any new medications you may start taking while on the program.

13.   Buy products that have nonfat or fat free labels.

14. You may divide your meals any way you like during a 16-hour period. But do not eat more than one allowed serving from a food group at one sitting.

15. We recommend eating your last meal at least 2 hours prior to going to bed.

16. If you are hungry, eat, but be sure you are hungry and not thirsty.

17. Plan menus in advance. Don't graze through the kitchen trying to find something to satisfy yourself.

18. Sit down to eat. Set a beautiful, pleasurable table, as if you were expecting a wonderful guest—yourself!

19. Don't do anything else while eating.

20. Eat consciously.

21. Do not change your eating habits dramatically. If your largest meal is lunch, keep it that way. If you're not a breakfast eater, you don't have to eat a large breakfast. However, do eat something in the morning!

22. Do not go longer than 4 hours during the day without eating something, even if it's just an apple.

23. Don't use diuretics or water pills unless specifically prescribed by your physician. Some natural recommendations can be found in the section on water and weight loss.

24. Be sure to weigh and measure foods carefully in the beginning until you can have a sense of the size and amount.

25. Cook fat free. Use a Teflon-coated pan or PAM cooking spray.

26. For constipation, some natural recommendations can be found in the section on weight loss interruptions.

27. Please notify the nurse of any medically related problems.

DAILY DIET PLAN

THE FOLLOWING PAGES LIST THE FOODS
ALLOWED ON THE DAILY DIET PLAN
BEGINNING ON
THE **THIRD DAY** OF THE PROGRAM.

A SIMPLE FORMULA TO HELP YOU
REMEMBER THE DIET PLAN IS:

EACH DAY:

TWO PROTEINS

TWO VEGETABLES

TWO BREADS (FIBERS)

TWO FRUITS

ONE EXTRA (see diet)

PROTEINS
1 - 6 oz. serving twice a day
(unless once a week is indicated)

1. Vary your selections
2. Fat-free cooking: Trim all visible fat
3. Broil, bake, barbecue, grill, or steam
4. Portions should be approximately 4 oz. servings (weigh portions before cooking)
5. Each serving should be a minimum of 3 hours apart (do not combine your daily portions; 4 oz. per meal)
6. Eat protein foods with vegetables (lightly cooked or raw)

*BEANS: *Once a week:* 1 cup of lentils, black beans, lima, navy, black-eyed peas (count also as one bread serving); do not cook with any meats or fats

BEEF: *Once a week:* eye of round or top round—lean, skinned, and fat trimmed; Healthy Choice ground beef only!

BEEF HEART: *Once a week:* 1 - 4 oz. serving

*CHEESE: *Once a week:* 100% fat free 4 oz. *or* 1/2 cup of Farmers/Alpine Lace/Healthy Choice (no others)

CHICKEN: White (breast) meat only; skinned, boned or ground and lean

COLD CUTS: *Once a week:* 2 slices per serving; turkey breast, chicken breast, ham (98% fat free, Healthy Choice)

*COTTAGE CHEESE: *Once a week:* 1/2 cup of nonfat *or* 1% low fat

*EGGS: *1 serving:* 1 egg and 2 whites (limit 2 servings per week; if cholesterol is over 200, use egg substitutes

*EGG SUB: *1 serving* (equivalent of 2 eggs): Eggbeaters, Scramblers, Second Nature

64

FISH (White):	*Fresh Preferred:* Bass, butterfish, blue fish, catfish, cod, flounder, grouper, haddock, halibut, kingfish, mahimahi, monk, orange roughy, pollock, sea bass, sea bream-sunfish, shark, smelt, sole, sturgeon, surimi (artificial crab, shrimp, and lobster), swordfish
FOWL:	Duck, pheasant, quail, squab, dove (all skinned)
HOT DOGS:	*Once a week:* 1 Healthy Choice Jumbo Franks *or* Hormel Light & Lean
***LENTILS/NAVY:**	*Once a week:* 1 cup (count as 1 protein serving and 2 bread servings)
LIVER:	*Once a week:* Calf or chicken (high in cholesterol)
***LOMA LINDA :**	*Once a week:* 1 patty of Dinner Cuts *or* 2 tbsp. Sandwich Spread *or* 4 pieces Tender Bits *or* 1/2 cup Vegeburger
PORK:	*Once a week:* Tenderloin only, 4 oz., fat trimmed
***PROTEIN POWDERS:**	You may use one drink per day for replacement of one meal if necessary
SEAFOOD:	Scallops, clams, mussels, oysters
SHELLFISH:	Crab, lobster, shrimp, prawns, clams, mussels, scallops, oysters (raw or steamed), 5-6 count as 1 protein
***SOYBEAN CURD:**	*Once a week:* 4 oz. *or* 1/2 cup
SURIMI:	*Once a week:* 4 oz. artificial crab, shrimp, lobster, *or* scallops (high in sodium)
***TOFU:**	Soybean curd, 4 oz. *or* 1/2 cup

TUNA:	4 oz., water-packed only
TURKEY:	Breast, skinned, white meat only, ground, lean
VEAL:	*Once a week:* 4 oz. of lean, all fat removed
VENISON:	Lean, all fat removed
***WORTHINGTON:**	*Once a week:* 1 patty Chicken Choplet *or* 2 oz. Soya meat
YOGURT:	*Once a week:* 1/2 cup, plain, nonfat, 4 oz.

*Vegetarian protein substitutes

VEGETABLES
1 serving, twice a day plus 1 raw snack

1. Vary your selection
2. Fresh preferred, raw or lightly cooked
3. Frozen or canned in low-sodium salt
4. If cooking, measure after cooking

1 CUP
Asparagus
Bamboo shoots
Brocoflower
Broccoli
Brussel sprouts (3-4 lg.)
Carrots (1 lg.)
Cauliflower
Chard
Chives
Jicama
Okra
Onions (white/yellow/red/green)
Parsley
Radishes (5-6)
Scallions
Snow peas
Tomato (1 med.)
Turnip
Watercress
Water chestnuts

1 - 1/2 CUPS
Alfalfa sprouts
Bean sprouts
Beets
Bok choy
Cabbage (red or white)
Chinese cabbage
Celery
Collard greens
Cucumber
Chicory
Endive
Escarole
Fennel
Kale
Kohlrabi
Mushrooms
Pepper (green or red)
Rhubarb
Spinach
Turnip greens
Zucchini

Lettuce *Unlimited :* iceberg, romaine, bibb, Boston

Tomato sauce *1/4 cup:* low sodium, no sugar

V-8 Juice *1 small can:* regular *or* tangy (low sodium)

ONCE A WEEK

Corn *1 medium:* fresh ear (yellow or white) *or* *3/4 cup* canned

Green beans *3/4 cup*

Peas *3/4 cup*

Squash *3/4 cup:* yellow, crookneck, acorn, scallop, spaghetti

Sweet potato or yam *1 medium*

CARBOHYDRATES
(Complex carbohydrates/fiber)
1 serving, twice a day

1. Vary your selection
2. Do not use butter or margarine
4. No breads or bagels with raisins
5. No croissants or tortilla chips

BAGEL: *1:* plain, egg, or onion (not flavored)

BARLEY: *1 cup:* cooked

BREAD or TOAST: *1 slice:* bran, cracked wheat, pumpernickel, french, sourdough, stone-ground, rye, Mal Sovit, Roman Meal Lite, Less Bread, *or* a low-calorie or lite bread

BREADSTICK: *1:* not flavored

BULGUR: *1 cup:* cooked; *1/2 cup:* wheat germ; *2-3 tbsp.:* unprocessed bran

BUNS: *1 bun:* hot dog *or* hamburger, counts as 2 bread servings (whole wheat preferred)

CEREAL, COLD : *1 cup:* with 1/2 cup skim or non-fat milk; no fruit, nuts, or raisins; *All Bran w/extra fiber, *Fiber One, Shredded Wheat 'N Bran, Shredded Wheat, Nutri-Grain, Wheat (Kellogg's) Bran Flake, Bran Chex, Wheat Chex, Total (whole wheat), Nutri-Grain; barley, rye or wheat, Mueslix 5-grain, Puffed Wheat or Rice, *or 1 cup* puffed kashi (* Indicates highest fiber)

CEREAL HOT: *1 cup:* cooked with 1/2 cup skim or non-fat milk; no fruit, nuts, or raisins; Quaker Old Fashioned Oats, Roman Meal Old Fashion (plain), Cream of Wheat, Farina, Wheat Hearts, Wheatena

68

CRACKERS:	***Limit 5 of one kind:*** Triscuits (low salt), Wheat 'N Bran, Krispy Low saltines, Waverly (low salt), Hi-Ho Whole Wheat, Premium low-salt saltines, Wheatsworth or Stoneground
CRACKER BREAD:	***Limit 3:*** Ak Mak, Wasa extra crisp, Crisp Bakes, Bran A Crisp, RyKrisp, Finn Crisp,
MELBA TOAST:	***2 slices***
MUFFINS:	***None***
PASTA:	***1 cup:*** cooked
PITA BREAD:	***1 large or 1/2 small:*** pita bread *or* pocket (whole wheat preferred)
POPCORN:	***3 cups:*** Light, non-flavored, microwave or air popped, "lite-salt" with no butter or salt (flavor with any Molly McButters)
POPCORN CAKE: (RICE CAKE)	***1 large cake:*** any brand, plain; any flavor, fat-free
TORTILLA:	***1 6-inch:*** corn or flour (cannot be made with lard)
WHEAT BRAN:	***1/2 cup:*** Wheat Bran Arrowhead Mills *or* Health Valley

ONE SERVING, ONCE A WEEK

PASTA: (EGG NOODLES)	***1/2 cup:*** cooked, whole wheat *or* spinach preferred
PASTA SAUCE:	***1/2 cup or 4 oz.:*** count as one vegetable serving, Healthy Choice spaghetti sauce
POTATO:	***1 medium:*** baked or boiled (red, new, or Idaho)
RICE:	***1 cup:*** cooked brown, white, or jasmine (brown preferred), no flavored unless listed; Pritikin Pilaf *or* Hains Three Grain Herb

FRUIT
SIMPLE CARBOHYDRATES/FIBER

1 serving, twice a day

1. Vary your selection
2. Fresh fruit preferred
3. No frozen fruit, fruit juices, fruit packed in light or heavy syrup, dried fruit rolls or bars

FRESH FRUIT:

Small fruit	2-1/2
Medium fruit	1-1/2
Large fruit	1
Bowl	1

APPLE: 1 large or 2 medium

APPLESAUCE: 3/4 cup of fresh *or* no sugar added *or* diet

APRICOTS: 3 medium *or* 3/4 cup of water packed

CANTALOUPE: 1/2 slice medium-size melon *or* 3/4 cup, fresh only

CASABA: 1 cup

CRANBERRY: 1 cup fresh only, no sugar added

GRAPEFRUIT: 1/2 of a small grapefruit

HONEYDEW: 3/4 cup

KIWI: 1 medium

MANGO: 1/2 slice or 3/4 cup

NECTARINE: 1 medium

ORANGE: 1 medium

PAPAYA: 1/2 slice

PEACH: 1 medium *or* 1/2 cup water packed

PEAR 2 medium *or* 1 cup water packed

PEACH:	1 large *or* 3/4 cup water packed
PINEAPPLE:	1 cup *or* 5 oz. of fresh (no canned)
POMEGRANATE:	1 medium
RHUBARB:	1-1/2 cups
STRAWBERRIES:	10 large berries *or* 3/4 cup fresh or frozen
TANGERINE:	1 medium
WATERMELON:	1-1/2 cup

ONCE A WEEK

BANANA:	1 medium
BERRIES:	3/4 cup fresh or frozen; blackberries, blueberries, boysenberries, gooseberries, raspberries
PLUM:	1 medium

*'Whatever you are afraid to do now
is the very thing you need to do next.'*

LIQUIDS

WATER IS ONE OF THE
MOST IMPORTANT PARTS OF THIS DIET!

1. Do not substitute or count other liquids as water
2. 2 quarts minimum per day
3. 3 quarts of water per day are preferable and recommended
4. Do not exceed 1 gallon (4 quarts) of water per day
5. No cream or cream substitutes

COFFEE: *Try to limit;* regular, Tasters Choice, no flavored instants

COFFEE (Decaf): *Unlimited* (water processed preferred)

CLUB SODA: *Unlimited*

CRYSTAL LIGHT: *2 - 8 oz.* glasses sugar free per day

DIET SODA: *Unlimited , 1 calorie or less;* caffeine free preferred

DIET TONIC: *Unlimited*

MILK: *1 teaspoon per cup:* skim (nonfat) milk for tea or coffee (powdered milk is o.k.)

MINERAL WATERS: *Unlimited:* nonflavored; Calistoga, Evian, Perrier, Vittel, Volvic

SANKA/POSTUM: *Unlimited*

SELTZER: *Unlimited:* salt free, diet only, no flavors, New York Seltzer

TEA (REGULAR): *Limited:* 2 cups if it has caffeine

TEA (HERBAL): *Unlimited:* all flavors

TEA (ICED): *Unlimited:* Fresh brewed herbal, sun tea, diet instants, sugar free

CONDIMENTS

DAILY

BOUILLON BROTH:	*1/4 cup:* low sodium
BUTTER:	*Unlimited:* Molly McButter (dry butter seasoning), Butter Buds
CATSUP:	*2 teaspoons:* Heinz light only
CONSOMME:	*1/4 cup:* low sodium
COOKING SPRAY:	PAM, fat free or butter flavored
COOKING WINE:	*1 tablespoon:* rice or cider vinegar (in place of wine)
HORSERADISH:	*1 tablespoon*
JUICES:	*2 tablespoons:* juice of a fresh lemon/lime/orange
KIKKOMAN:	*1 tablespoon:* "Lite" soy sauce
MILK:	*2 tablespoon:* Skim, nonfat
MAYONNAISE:	*2 tablespoons:* Kraft Free
MUSTARD:	*1 tablespoon:* regular, Dijon
PARMESAN CHEESE:	*1 tablespoon*
RELISH:	*1 teaspoon:* pickle relish only; no pickles
SALAD DRESSING:	*2 tablespoons :* All flavors Kraft Free (fat free), Good Seasons fat free; no other light or reduced-calorie salad dressing; *or* **2 tbsp.** Estee or Dia-Mel, all flavors
SALSA:	*2 tablespoons:* picante
SUGAR:	*Sparingly:* Sweet-N-Low, Sugar Twin, Nutra-Sweet, or Equal
TABASCO SAUCE:	*1 teaspoon*
TACO SAUCE:	*2 tablespoons*
WORCESTERSHIRE:	*1 teaspoon*

SEASONINGS

DAILY

BUTTER: Molly McButter dry butter seasoning

GARLIC: *1 clove*

MRS. DASH: *Unlimited*

PARSLEY PATCH: *1 teaspoon*

PEPPER: *Unlimited:* regular or lemon pepper

SALT: *Moderation:* Morton's Lite

SPIKE: *1 teaspoon*

VEGE-SAL: *1 teaspoon*

VEGEIT: *1 teaspoon*

LIMIT TO 2 TEASPOONS

ALL SEASONINGS: fresh, dried, or powdered; sweet basil, tarragon leaves, ginger, bay leaves, cinnamon, curry, dill, oregano, paprika, nutmeg, etc.

NATURAL GOURMET SEASONINGS:
no salt, sugar, or monosodium glutamate (MSG)

"Eat to live — don't live to eat!"

74

MISCELLANEOUS EXTRAS

DAILY

BREATH MINTS:	*2 a day:* sugarless only
COOL WHIP:	*1 tablespoon:* Light, nondairy
D-ZERTA:	*1 cup:* made as directed
GUM:	*2 sticks*, sugarless
JELL-O GELATIN:	*1 cup:* Jell-O, sugar-free
JELL-O PUDDING:	*1/2 cup:* sugar-free, made with nonfat skim milk
JELLY/JAM:	*2 teaspoons:* Estee, Dia-mel or Smuckers light, all natural, no sugar
POPSICLE:	*1* sugar-free Popsicle or Crystal Light brand (no juice or fruit bars)
SALSA:	*2 tablespoons*
SOUR CREAM:	*1 teaspoon:* imitation, nonfat (Light N' Lively-Free)
SWEETENERS:	*Unlimited:* Nutra Sweet or Equal preferred; Sweet-N-Low, Sugar Twin acceptable
TACO SAUCE:	*2 tablespoons:* Ortega
YOGURT:	*1 - 5 oz.:* regular, frozen, nonfat (no toppings)

MEASUREMENTS:

4 oz. = 1/4 pound

4 fluid oz. = 1/2 cup

8 fluid oz. = 1 cup

No anger can be provoked
Which does not lie sleeping in my breast—

Nor fear aroused
Which is not coiled slumbering in my pits.

No dark emotion can be awakened in me
That does not already lie sleeping
In the recesses of my Being.

And to that committed soul
Who disturbs my apparent peaceful veneer

I owe Acknowledgment, Gratitude
and Response-Ability

It is my promise as an Awake Being
To own the emotions that others urge to the light

And rather than loose them
on my undeserving friends
Where they would harm us all,

I shall offer them up to the water,
the wind and the Earth,
Where their energies can be discharged
To more loving purposes

—Roseanna, 1988

When caffeine was taken together with physical activity, the thermogenic effect was enhanced. The mechanism by which caffeine exerts this fat-burning effect is thought to be associated with the thermogenic cori cycle. This is where glycogen and glucose are converted to lactate in fat and muscle tissue. Lactate then triggers thermogenic processes in the liver.

For an adult, caffeine in small doses (50 mg. to 200 mg., no more than three times a day) appears to have few harmful effects. More than this, however, may often cause symptoms ranging in severity from nervousness to possible increased risk for developing degenerative diseases. When caffeine intake is compared to body weight, one caffeinated soft drink to a 30-pound child is equivalent to five cups of coffee to a 150-pound adult. The caffeine content of coffee and tea increase with prolonged steeping time and increased strength of the brew.

Caffeine is habit forming, and research shows that indeed it could be addictive. Depression, headaches, irritability, and lethargy are possible symptoms of caffeine withdrawal.

Throughout the world, there are at least 117 plants known to stimulate the central nervous system (CNS), which, in turn, may result in an increased metabolic rate and subsequent weight loss. Other herbs may act as stimulants through biochemical pathways operating outside of CNS channels. Plants that energize human systems bring about increased metabolic rates and result in weight loss and increased physical stamina. Some of these herbs are cayenne, damiana, ginseng, and schisandra.

"Health is a lack of dis-ease."

THE PLATEAU DIET

Please read the section entitled "The Plateau"
before you use this plateau diet.

A "plateau" with regard to this diet may last from four or five days to a week. The first one frequently occurs during the third or fourth week. This is a common aspect at some point in any weight loss program and is usually synonymous with a previous "set weight." It is very individual in time and duration.

A plateau does not mean you are not responding to treatment. However, if after three or four days you get impatient and discouraged you can stimulate the weight loss by having an "apple day."

Unless your weight has been stationary *at least* three days without dietary error, you will not be eligible for the apple day diet.

The apple day should produce a loss of weight on the following day.

1.   An apple day begins with the beginning of the day and continues until the beginning of the next day.

2.   You may eat up to eight medium-size apples whenever you feel the desire to eat.

3.   No other foods are allowed.

4.   You do not have to eat all eight apples.

5.   Four small cantaloupes may be *substituted* for the eight apples.

6.   It will not be necessary on this day to drink the full amount of your daily water requirement. Drink only what you wish.

DO NOT USE THIS PLATEAU DIET
FOR MORE THAN ONE DAY AT A TIME!

THE SPECIAL DIET*

**These special instructions
are only to be used and approved by
your physician in addition to the regular diet.**

1.   Limit fruit.

2.   Concentrate on green vegetables: **200–250** calories daily from root vegetables, raw only.

3.   Do not use table salt.

4.   Drink only sodium-free and caffeine-free diet drinks.

5.   Three equal meals of a minimum of **350** calories each

6.   If you are taking insulin, you *must not* skip meals.

7.   Drink **10** oz. of liquid every **2** hours while awake.

8.   **Consult your physician immediately if you are not clear about these particular guidelines.**

9.   Any other guidelines specific to you will be given by your physician.

***For use only by people with borderline diabetes,
glucose intolerance, or morbid obesity.**

Write down any instructions below:

DAILY WEIGHT LOSS RECORD

DATE	WEIGHT	DATE	WEIGHT

82

DAILY INCH LOSS RECORD

DATE:____BUST:____WAIST:_____ABDOMEN:____ HIPS:____

DATE:____BUST:____WAIST: ____ ABDOMEN:_____HIPS:____

DATE: ____BUST:____ WAIST: ____ABDOMEN: ____HIPS: ____

DATE: ____BUST:____WAIST: ____ABDOMEN: ____HIPS: ____

DATE: ____BUST:____WAIST: ____ABDOMEN: ____HIPS: ____

DATE: ____BUST:____WAIST: ____ABDOMEN: ____HIPS:____

DATE: ____BUST:____WAIST: ____ABDOMEN: ____HIPS:____

DATE: ____BUST:____WAIST: ____ABDOMEN: ____HIPS:____

DATE: ____BUST:____WAIST: ____ABDOMEN: ____HIPS:____

DATE:____BUST:____ WAIST: ____ABDOMEN: ____HIPS: ____

DATE: ____BUST:____WAIST: ____ABDOMEN: ____HIPS: ____

DATE: ____BUST:____WAIST: ____ABDOMEN: ____HIPS:____

DATE: ____BUST:____WAIST: ____ABDOMEN: ____HIPS: ____

JENNY

My niece started gaining weight in junior high school by the time she graduated she weight 150 pounds

I went to San Francisco for her graduation and could tell by the way she walked and avoided any eye contact that the weight problem was effecting her emotionally as well as physically. I talked with her that evening and we decided that she would come home with me and start her on the program as soon as she could completed her lab and physical. Her parents agreed and we left with high hopes.

Jenny began her program with enthusiasm. She went to the clinic every day and helped with the filing and paperwork. When our receptionist took her vacation Jenny filled in for her.

She lost fifteen pounds the first month and set her goal to lose fifteen more. In four more weeks she had reached her goal. We went to a hair stylist and she got a great hair cut and brightened her hair color to a beautiful auburn shade. Our next trip was to get her something new to wear because none of her old clothes fit her as she had dropped three dress sizes. She hadn't seen any of her family during her stay.

We left for San Francisco with great expectations. Her parents live in a typical Bay area home with a garage on the first level and the living area above. As we pulled up in front of the house we could see her parents in front of the window waiting for us. Jenny had selected an emerald green pant suit and took great care in applying her make-up. She looked entirely different than the person I had left with. Her mother came down the stairs to greet us and called out to me and asking where Jenny was. Jenny ran up to her with a big hug and when her mother realized who it was, we all had a good cry. Her whole family expressed their amazement at her transformation. Naturally this is one of the most gratifying experiences, as it involves someone so close.

*"I control my life absolutely.
I am stepping away from old habits."*

—Stuart Wilde

CHAPTER SIX

The Work Out

GOOD HEALTH

Good health is something we can "choose" to have by consciously deciding to do those things that support well being.

It also involves taking responsibility for wellness and not blaming how we feel on our family, doctors, environment, friends, or circumstances.

Our level of health, right this moment, is a result of the countless choices we have made regarding the foods we select, the exercise we get, and the thoughts we think.

At any moment, we can choose differently. Where this new "choice" making begins, I believe, is with appreciating and respecting our marvelous bodies. The body is indeed a miracle of divine creation, and the more I study about the body, the more I am amazed at how beautifully it is designed.

In terms of a cold scientific analysis, the body might be regarded as being two-thirds water, plus carbon, calcium, and other chemicals worth just a few dollars (even at the inflated prices).

Right now, just as we are sitting, standing, or lying down, our bodies are performing amazing feats of engineering, chemistry, and physics that no engine designed by woman or man can duplicate.

What's more, the body improves with use. For example, the more stress we put on our bodies through physical exercise, the stronger our bones and muscles will become and the more efficiently the body will function.

Clearly the body is fantastic and deserves respect and appreciation.

— From a "Unity" article by Susan Smith Jones

THE DIET WARS:
WHEN YOUR BODY FIGHTS BACK

We've all heard stories about people who lose 100 pounds on a liquid diet, only to regain 150.

Now researchers believe they have a clue to why this happens. According to a recent study in the *New England Journal of Medicine,* the culprit may be an enzyme called lipoprotein lipase that facilitates the storage of fat.

When obese subjects lose a lot of weight, researchers found, this enzyme becomes much more active, and the heavier the dieters are to begin with, the more active the enzyme becomes. Enzyme overactivity may also explain why the formerly fat often battle intense food cravings: Scientists theorize that lipoprotein lipase sends appetite-regulating signals to the brain. Moderately overweight people who lose 20 or 30 pounds probably shouldn't blame lipoprotein lipase if fat comes back, however, says Phillip Kern, the head researcher and an endocrinologist at Cedars-Sinai Medical Center in Los Angeles. Enzyme levels seem to rise only in men and women who have been extremely obese.

"Maturity consists of no longer taking one's self seriously."

88

THE EXERCISE CONNECTION

In a diet program, the importance of exercise can't be ignored. As a matter of fact, in general health or any diet, exercise is an inseparable and integral aspect. Diet increases the benefits of exercise and vice versa.

In a primitive or agrarian society, exercise probably wasn't a problem. People got their daily exercise naturally, mainly in their daily work. Our sedentary lifestyles (automobiles, elevators, desk jobs) make some sort of exercise routine vital for health.

Muscles are made to be exercised. It's their way of receiving new nutrients and discarding waste products. Exercise moves the lymphatic system. The temporary increase in body temperature kills (pasteurizes) viruses and bacteria, making exercise an important immune system support.

Strive to have a protein/vegetable meal eaten early in the day. That way, late afternoon to early evenings become the most productive time for strenuous exercise.

It takes approximately 8 hours for proteins to be digested, assimilated, humanized by the liver, and made available to the cells, provided the liver is in good working order. The proteins eaten early in the day are already assimilated by evening and they are ready to build and rebuild tissues. Exercise is essential to move proteins out of the lymphatic system into the cells where they can rebuild and renew life at the cellular level.

Remember that upper-body exercise is as important as lower-body exercise. The arms move the lymphatic system and work the internal organs. Swimming and moving the arms through water is a particularly good form of exercise that works both upper and lower halves of the body.

Brisk walking and stretching shortly after awakening raise the basal metabolism and make for an alert, energetic day. Strenuous workouts and thorough exercise programs are best 8-10 hours after breakfast.

The program puts a high emphasis on exercise for not only the more visible benefits such as enhanced mental, physical, and emotional well-being, improved physical stamina, relief of tension and stress, improved circulation, and improved muscle tone, but also for other, not-so-obvious reasons.

Regular and moderate exercise works with your body to increase your basal metabolic rate and the rate of fat calorie burning. They also lower and reduce the appetite and will help you in maintaining your desired weight.

Aerobic Exercise

The exercise must be aerobic. By aerobic, we mean you must keep it steady (nonstop) and continuous for a minimum of 20 minutes. You must bring your heart rate to a specific range and hold this heart rate for a 20-minute period.

Nonaerobic sports, such as racquetball or tennis, will not hold your heart rate at a steady level for a determined time because they are not steady and do not sustain maximum heart rates.

The heart rate determined for you is calculated to bring your heart to approximately 70% of maximum.

If you do two sets of 10-minute exercises you will not raise your metabolic rate or lower your set weight.

Time and Duration

You must exercise a minimum of 3-4 days per week, 30 minutes per day. Ten minutes of the exercise should be for warm-up and cool-down. If you exercise 2 days a week or less you lose the desired benefits. If you exercise 3-4 days a week you maintain your muscle tone, chemistry, metabolic rate and fat-burning capacity.

If you exercise 5-6 days per week you will improve your muscle tone, alter your body chemistry, and increase your metabolic rate and fat calorie burning rate.

More importantly, exercising 5 days per week at a given heart rate for a given duration not only assures these benefits, but will continue to be effective for up to 24 hours after you stop exercising, even while you're sleeping.

As an example, if it's recommended that you bring your target heart rate to between 110 and 120, you will want to maintain a pulse of 11-12 beats in a six-second period. This is where you want to keep your heart rate for the 20-minute aerobic period. If it is too high, slow down.

Listen to your body! You will not benefit from your exercise by pushing yourself too hard. For your own safety and to achieve optimal results, keep within your target heart rate.

Key Points To Remember

1. Aerobic exercise is steady and nonstop.

2. Hold your heart rate at the prescribed level for 20 minutes.

3. Always monitor your pulse.

4. Always warm up and cool down.

5. Duration, not intensity, is the goal (minimum of 5 days per week, 30 minutes per day).

6. Keep a record of your progress.

7. Choose an exercise you enjoy.

8. If you start getting bored, change exercises.

9. Use variety in exercises so that each of the muscle groups gets a workout.

10. At no time should your heart rate exceed 80% of your maximum heart rate.

11. Do not confuse your target heart rate with your maximum heart rate.

Warm-up and Cool-down

This is a must in your exercise program to prevent injury and undue strain on the muscles. Remember, your heart is a muscle too.

Always warm up before you exercise; include this as part of the aerobic routine. When the routine is over, cool down, stretch, and continue to do deep breathing to supply oxygen to the muscle tissues. Never stretch beyond your capability, either before or after exercise.

Even if you haven't exercised in years you can begin with moderate to brisk walking. Make sure the exercise is continuous, steady, and reaches your prescribed target heart rate for 20 minutes.

It is not the intensity of the exercise but the gradual, progressive, and sustained aerobic exercise that gives you optimal results.

Your target heart rate:_____

Pulse Monitoring

To determine that you're getting your heart to your prescribed THR, you need to monitor your pulse. Place your second and third fingers over your wrist, palm side up, just below the thumb, until you can feel your pulse and count it. Count the number of beats for 6 seconds and add a zero to the number. This is your pulse or heart rate; you may find it easier to get an accurate pulse in your neck. Ask your health instructor or your doctor or nurse to demonstrate the carotid pulse technique.

Take your heart rate before exercising or when getting up in the morning. You will get a pulse of approximately 70-80 (or 7-8 beats in a 6-second period), which is your resting heart rate (RHR).

*"Health is the willingness
to use your body with love".*

SUGGESTED AEROBIC EXERCISES

Aerobic dancing
Backpacking
Basketball
Chairstepping
Cross-country skiing
Cycling outdoors
Dancing
Ice skating
Jumping jacks
Jumping rope
Mini-trampoline (rebounder)

Race walking
Roller skating
Rowing
Running in place
Running or jogging
Stair climbing
Stationary bicycling
Sparring or boxing
Swimming
Walking or brisk
walking

CLASS LEVEL:_____   TIME: _____

HEART RATE: _____ 30 DAYS: _____ 60 DAYS: _____

	REST	WORKING	RECOVERY
MONDAY:			
TUESDAY:			
WEDNESDAY:			
THURSDAY:			
FRIDAY:			
SATURDAY:			
SUNDAY:			

PROGRAM EXERCISE RECORD

Best types of exercise for weight control: Continuous aerobic;
walking, stationary cycling, swimming, pool walking, and rowing
Frequency: Minimum of 3 days per week, 5 days per week
maximum
Duration: Build up to 20 minutes to start; 60 minutes goal of
continuous aerobic activity
Each exercise session: 5–10 minutes warm-up, 20 minutes
aerobic exercise, 5–10 minutes cool-down

Goals				Actual						
WEEK	TYPE	FREQUENCY	DURATION	S	M	T	W	T	F	S

WHAT IS A WORKOUT?

A workout is 25% perspiration and 75% determination. Stated another way, it is one part physical exertion and three parts self-discipline. Doing it is easy once you get started. A workout makes you better today than you were yesterday. It strengthens the body, relaxes the mind and toughens the spirit. When you work out regularly, your problems diminish and your confidence grows. A workout is a personal triumph over laziness and procrastination. It is the badge of a winner. The mark of an organized, goal-oriented person who has taken charge of his, or her, destiny. A workout is a wise use of time and an investment in excellence. It is a way of preparing for life's challenges and proving to yourself that you have what it takes to do what is necessary. A workout is a key that helps unlock the door to opportunity and success. Hidden within each of us is an extraordinary force. Physical and mental fitness are the triggers that can release it. A workout is a form of rebirth. When you finish a good workout, you don't simply feel better—you feel better about yourself!

—George Allen

In this statement,
nutritionist and philosopher **Paul Bragg**
offers us a vivid idea
of just how wonderful the body really is:

'Now stop and think!

The Creator has presented you with

the world's most wonderful machine —

your own body.

This miracle·machine has its own

nonstop motor (the heart),

its own fueling system (the digestive tract),

its own filtration system (kidneys),

its own temperature control (sweat glands),

and so on. Indeed, this most remarkable

contrivance even has the power

to reproduce itself."

"Truth is my friend"

· Stuart Wilde

CHAPTER SEVEN

Staying Out

DON'T BE AFRAID TO FAIL

You've failed many times, although you may not remember.

You fell down the first time you tried to walk.

You almost drowned the first time you tried to swim.

Did you hit the ball the first time you swung a bat?

Heavy hitters who hit the most home runs, also strike out a lot.

R.H. Macy failed seven times before his New York store caught on.

Novelist J. Creasey got 753 rejection slips before his 564 books.

Babe Ruth struck out 1,330 times; he also hit 714 home runs.

How many times did you try to quit smoking?

Did ice skating come naturally?

Riding a bicycle was easy, after the hundredth time.

How many different types of diets have you gone on?

Don't worry about failure . . .

Just do it!

MAINTENANCE

As Albert Einstein taught us, matter and energy are differentiated principally by form. Your body is a form of energy slowed down to assume the appearance of matter. And the mind directs the energy that determines the form.

You do have the power to create the form you desire to live in. You may choose to change your form by losing weight, but first you must know that you don't have to be slender to be acceptable to others. While it is true that fat people can create negative reactions, even hostility, in others, the important point, as this entire book emphasizes, is not how others view you but *how you view yourself.* If you are truly comfortable with your form, fine. For whatever your choice, you are complete.

Long-term "Natural" Weight

You will spend a number of weeks learning new habits and behaviors. As you approach your desired weight, you need to begin thinking of your maintenance plan and how to maintain your new "natural" weight.

Remember, it is much easier to gain unwanted pounds than it is to lose them. The maintenance program is as important as the weight loss program. Once there, you can maintain your ideal weight by simply applying your acquired knowledge and eating habits and expanding on them.

An important factor is getting a head start on a successful maintenance program and keeping in mind how crucial the first four weeks are. This is when your body needs to adjust to the new "set weight." It is also the time when it is much easier to gain your weight back.

After the initial program, it is recommended that you go in at least once a month to your doctor's office. Have the nurse weigh you, check your blood pressure, and take measurements. In this way, you are able to monitor your weight. If they have any objections to supporting you in this way, look for another physician that will.

One of the best methods of maintaining your weight loss is very simple, but it must become a way of life for you to succeed.

100

When you are through with your program and have achieved your natural goal weight, you must weigh yourself every morning. As long as you are within 2 pounds of that weight, you are fine. The first morning that you discover you are more than 2 pounds over your natural new weight, you must eat only one meal that day.

We suggest a broiled or baked chicken breast (boned and skinned) and a sliced tomato. This can be eaten at any time during the day, but it must be the only meal you eat. The next morning, when you weigh, you will discover that you have returned to your original weight. By doing this each time, you will never lose control of your weight again.

Two other options for maintaining are found under "A One-Day Fast" and "The Plateau Diet."

As long as you decide ahead of time that you will faithfully weigh every day, and have decided which of the options you prefer, the only thing left to do is to . . . **JUST DO IT!**

*"Deep within you
is everything that is natural and perfect,
it only waits upon you
to allow it to come through
and into the world."*

REASONS TO MAINTAIN MY PRESENT WEIGHT

Write down reasons why you want to keep your weight off. These will be your motivators for weight maintenance. Make sure these are personal reasons, not what you think society or your significant others want.

Anytime you need reinforcement or support, refer back to this list. Keep adding to your list as you continue to reinforce your reasons to maintain at your natural weight.

1. _____

2. _____

3. _____

4. _____

5. _____

6. _____

7. _____

8. _____

9. _____

10. _____

THE INFAMOUS REPEATER

Repeated dieting leads to greater difficulty in losing weight, greater efficiency in gaining weight, and a tendency to overeat once food becomes available.

Many of you will retain water after you stop an inappropriate diet because your bodies overcompensate and retain excessive water in and between the cells. With this "refeeding edema," dieters suffer from chronic swelling. You can read more about this in the water retention section of this book.

Moreover, the dieter often becomes confused and depressed from continuing to make a commitment that ends up in yet another failure. Despite adherence to a low-calorie diet plan, a protein fasting, or a supplemental diet, you can actually end up gaining weight instead of losing it.

Frequent dieting also lowers the metabolic rate (the number of calories you burn to support normal body functions). With all this taken into consideration, is it any wonder that at least half or more of the adult population diets, and that 70% of those people will be "quick" or "fad" weight loss repeaters?

Any weight problem, whether it's big or small, can do more than just affect your appearance. Your outlook and attitude on life are affected as well. Being overweight by as little as 10–20 pounds can often undermine a person's sense of confidence and self-worth.

Another observed result of dieting is that when people go on low-calorie diets, they lose their appetites. As long as people remain on their diets, they're okay, but as soon as they try to maintain their desired weight, their problems begin again.

When you go on a maintenance program, not only do you regain water and regain fat more readily because your metabolic rate is lower, but in addition your appetite becomes stimulated by food, so you're more likely to overeat. This becomes the epidemic of inappropriate dieting.

People can't expect to alter their normal biology by starving. The evidence shows that repeated dieting—taking weight off and putting it back on again and again—is becoming an all-too-common phenomenon. More than being extremely frustrating for the "yo-yo" dieter, recent studies suggest that these repeated bouts of weight loss and gain make weight control more difficult and contribute to health risks.

Your maintenance program is just as important for you as the weight loss program itself. Returning to your doctor's office periodically can allow you to be monitored and will give you that added support and the necessary assurance that you will receive assistance if problems arise.

"Whatever you are trying to avoid
won't go away—
it will continue to find you
until you are willing to confront it."

MAINTAINING MAINTENANCE˜

Tell yourself the truth!
It's not just a diet, it's an entire lifestyle.
Set realistic, comfortable goals.
Be light-hearted.
Don't dwell on your weaknesses and setbacks. Go forward.
Breathe (take deep, slow, full cleansing breaths) when stressed.
Anticipate difficult situations. Have a game plan.
Imagine your "naturally slender" self right now! Don't accept less.
Accept where you are now. Live in the moment!
Discover the power of writing down your experiences.
Listen to your body's signals for "hunger" and "satisfaction."
Are you hungry for "nourishment" or hungry for "nurturing"?
Rearrange your environment to please and nurture yourself.
Let go of the need to save, please, or caretake others.
Please yourself.
Be willing to know the truth.
Learn to say "yes." Learn to say "no."
Practice self-forgiveness to stop a lapse from becoming a relapse.
Nurture yourself in some way every day for the rest of your life.
Look yourself in the eyes in a mirror for a full 5 minutes each day.
Feel your feelings. Be with your feelings. Express your feelings.
If you're angry. . . be angry. Be with your anger. It's part of you too.
Turn mistakes into learning experiences rather than giving up.
Be still and listen.
Make conscious choices!
Visualize success.
What would it look like to weigh less?
Confront the stress in your life and eliminate it.
Embrace your fears.
Develop relationships and activities that enrich and relax your life.
Create reality yourself—don't stand and watch it go by.
Accept yourself only the way you want to be.
Love your body just as it is—as it changes each day.
Exchange the word "challenge" for "problem."
Whatever you fear the most—do it first!
Take more risks.
Trust your body's feelings and signals.
Focus on what *is* in your life, not on what isn't.
Monitor your self-talk.
Release people and places that don't support and honor you.
Reclaim your power. Go for it!   *—Own your own life now!*

WEIGHT LOSS INTERRUPTION

Please be sure to inform your physician if any of the following should occur or if any illnesses, injuries, discomfort, or unusual circumstances arise during your program. Also, all the suggestions for products below should be approved by your physician prior to purchase.

NORMAL FLUCTUATION

It is very important to be aware of your own weight loss patterns. By this we mean that each individual has a different rate of weight loss and of metabolism.

You should fall into an average weight loss category. For example: 1/4 pound per day for women, 1/2 pound a day for men. *However, that does not mean that you will consistently lose that amount of weight every day!* You may lose 3 pounds on one day and 1 pound the next.

It is important to recognize your own weight loss pattern and that your average overall loss will not necessarily be the same as that of someone else. You must look at the overall picture. If you forget this important point, you may not show a weight loss on the scale yet actually feel lighter and be disappointed.

Often the proof is in the measurements, not in the pounds. A lot of people are losing inches and not pounds during certain periods of the program. Weight loss is not always accountable on the scale. It may be found on the measurement tape.

Remember to look at the overall picture and don't always put all the emphasis on the numbers. Have patience with yourself. You are making progress even if it doesn't show on the scales. You are focused, determined, and committed. Give yourself praise for how far you have come and trust that you are moving toward your natural weight.

Don't be discouraged! Give yourself time to get into a rhythm. What is normal for someone else is not necessarily normal for you. You will move into your own distinct pattern of weight loss. There are too many variables to pigeonhole any one particular "normal" for everyone. Also, your body periodically needs to stabilize itself.

You are making changes in your attitude and lifestyle and you have to expect some resistance from your body to keep it the old way. Make sure you put aside time to nurture yourself and your body. You both deserve some loving and quiet time for all the effort.

106

MENSTRUAL CYCLE

This type of interruption normally occurs a few days before and during the menstrual period and, in some women, at the time of ovulation. This is due to the natural hormonal changes and fluctuations, often accompanied by some degree of water retention. It is not considered an actual weight gain, per se, but an interruption in metabolism and elimination. Remember that it is a temporary situation. Don't resent it—just "flow" with it (small pun intended). *If you should become pregnant during the treatment, notify your physician and discontinue the program immediately.*

CONSTIPATION

If this tends to be a chronic problem, please notify your physician. This is the least likely cause for weight loss interruption. Prevention is the best treatment. Be sure to eat the bread and fiber portions as required and drink plenty of water.

Preventive: 1 tbsp. sugar-free Fiberall or sugar-free Metamucil, Swiss cress (herb), or psyllium fiber

Do not use Ex-lax or similar laxatives.

Suggestions: Atri-aloe-v 450 mg., 1 tablet daily (can be ordered from Atrium, Inc., P.O. Box 123 South Street, Coloma, WI 54930); glycerin or Dulcolax suppository or Colace or Surfax stool softeners
Do not take a strong laxative or enema without your physician's knowledge.
For hemorrhoids: Preparation H, Nupercainal cream, or Tucks pads

COLDS AND FLU

Force lots of liquids (preferably water)
Hot herbal teas
Natural, sugarless juices

SORE THROAT OR COUGH

Sugar-free cough syrup, limit as much as possible (i.e., Dimacol, Polytuss DM)
Gargle with warm salt water (sea salt)
Warm herbal teas with lemon
Warm water with fresh lemon
N'ICE sugarless throat lozenges
Vicks Vapo Rub on throat and chest

HYPERACIDITY
1 oz. Maalox or Mylanta or equivalent (low-sodium and sugar free;
one Tums or Calcitrel tablet as indicated (could contribute to
constipation)

CONGESTION
Nasal spray or drops, oral decongestants with antihistamine

LOSS OF APPETITE (MINIMAL REQUIREMENT)

PROTEIN:

4 oz. low-fat/skim cottage cheese
8 oz. low-sodium consommé/broth,
   prepared as directed
8 oz. low-sodium vegetable broth
1 poached or soft-boiled egg
8 oz. Pritikin soup

VEGETABLE:

6 oz. V-8 vegetable juice
6 oz. low-sodium vegetable juice
Steam or boil vegetables until soft, purée in
   blender with a small amount of mild
   seasoning

FRUIT:

1/2 cup sugar-free applesauce
Cantaloupe or ripe melon
Easily digestible fruit in the afternoon or evening
Sugar-free Jell-O

BREAD:

Toast, no butter
Low-salt crackers

SOCIAL AND BUSINESS ENGAGEMENTS

These days restaurants are very aware of the needs of health-conscious diners. Most of the time they will make every effort to fill your requests for specifics in preparing your meals any way you would like.

Ask your waiter to have the chef steam your selection without oils, butter, or salt. You may be pleasantly surprised that most restaurants are now offering several healthful choices on the menu to accommodate you and your selections.

SUGGESTIONS:

1.   Eat *before* you go to a function if you know that you will have a difficult and tempting time with the meal.

2.   Avoid going places where you can't make choices about what you want.

3.   Don't allow others to pressure you into eating something you don't want or need.

4.   Don't feel you have to clean your plate.

5.   Enjoy the occasion, conversation, and friends as much as the food.

6.   Don't set yourself up to fail by making excuses that you could have avoided.

7.   Discriminate about whom you go to lunches, parties, and functions with. Make sure they are willing to support you instead of making you feel deprived or guilty.

8.   Re-evaluate occasions that are based on food. Thanksgiving, Christmas, barbecues, and the like can all have more value than the food. Be creative and put more of your energies into other areas of the celebration. Try to put more emphasis on the relationships or the environment instead of spending all your time, effort, and money toward a 30-minute feast!

9.   Find out ahead of time if your host or hostess is be willing to

make you a special plate with only the healthful parts of the
meal to be served.

10.　Start looking at menus for items that respect your health and
your commitment to better well-being. A lot of restaurants
and food places are striving to bring a wider variety of choices
to the general public with regard to their health concerns. If
your favorite restaurant doesn't seem to offer you something
you feel would benefit you and others who are working on
weight issues, bring that to the manager's attention and see
if he or she would be willing to accommodate you with an
additional item or two on the menu. Remember, the restaurant
is there to *serve you* and is usually very receptive to your
requests.

11.　If you are about to eat something that is not on the diet, don't
look for excuses and try to justify what you are about to do.
Just make an aware, conscious choice that you are going to
eat what you want instead of what you are required to eat.
Then eat it! But don't spend 2 hours before and 24 hours
afterward feeling guilty. Just acknowledge that you are
making a choice and you may or may not have weight gain
consequences. It does not serve you to cheat or deny that you
are going to eat something that you want. No one is watching
you or waiting to see if you do or do not eat something that
you're not supposed to.

*You are the only one who is responsible for
what you do and what decisions you make.
It is your body and your decision!*

You are the one who wants an end result. However, if you choose to
eat off the diet (cheat) periodically, enjoy it. But don't spend the next
days wallowing in guilt and recrimination. Just do it and then get on
with your diet as you should.

Once you set up a denial process, you will eat just to defy anyone
(especially yourself) to tell you that you can't eat something. So don't
deny yourself if it's something that you really want or an occasion
that is really special.

Just make a conscious choice about what you are about to do and
then do it! Savor the moment, then forget about it, let it go, and get
on with life and your regular diet.

SOME SELECTION SUGGESTIONS

APPETIZERS

Raw vegetables
Sliced roast beef or turkey
Fresh fruit slices
Fruit drink with crushed ice (without alcohol)
Shrimp, crab, or lobster
Diet tonic water or low-sodium club soda
Diet 7-up with fresh fruit slices
Fresh water with a slice of lemon or lime

SOUP AND SALAD

Salad bars offer lots of variety (diet dressings)
Soups — bouillon or onion (no croutons, cheese, or cream
soups)

MAIN COURSES

Breakfast: poached egg on toast (no butter)
Sliced fruit salad
Chef or crab salad, low-fat cottage cheese
Green salad with tomato and diet dressing
Low-fat cottage cheese
Lean steak, prime rib, or roast beef
Chicken breast (skinned, no sauces)
Lobster or prawns

VEGETABLES

Many restaurants offer a vegetarian selection or steamed
vegetables. Leave off the butter or ask for an extra portion
in place of the rice or potato.

Alcohol is strictly forbidden while on this program, not only because of the calorie/carbohydrate content and lack of nutritional value, but also because a relatively small amount of alcohol will produce intoxication while on the program. Your system is much more sensitive to alcohol, and it will also cause a rapid weight gain out of proportion to the amount consumed. Alcohol is high in calories and carbohydrates. Under no circumstances are any medications to be mixed with alcohol.

HEALTH GUIDELINES

The National Heart, Lung and Blood Institute (NHLBI) has determined that there are five main controllable risk factors for coronary heart disease, this country's major health concern.

A risk factor is a habit, trait, or condition in a person that is associated with an increased chance (or risk) of developing a disease.

These five factors are:

1. excess body weight,
2. elevated blood cholesterol levels,
3. high blood pressure,
4. cigarette smoking, and
5. lack of physical exercise.

Any three of these risk factors combined may increase the risk of heart disease by a factor of 10 or more.

Our diet and program aim at not only supporting you to reach a normal and desired body weight, but also concurrently affect all of these factors to a large degree.

CHOLESTEROL

When you begin the program your lab results should indicate your serum (blood) cholesterol level.

The desirable range, according to the NHLBI, is a cholesterol reading of 200 mg. or less for anyone over the age of 30. Levels above 220 mg. place the individual in moderate to high risk.

By using our diet (which follows NHLBI guidelines) and lowering your weight, you will lower your cholesterol. Studies have shown that, as an example, if you lost 22 pounds you could expect your cholesterol level to drop 20 mg. If you cut your cholesterol by 25%, you cut your risk of heart attack in half. If your cholesterol level is elevated, your physician will want to recheck it in 6-8 weeks.

For most individuals, blood cholesterol can be lowered by eating *less saturated fat.* Key points to remember are:

Cholesterol is found only in animal products (organ meats, egg yolks, meat, butter, and cheese).

Saturated fat is found mostly in animal products and some vegetable oils (cocoa fat, chocolates, and shortenings).

Vegetables, fruits, cereal grains, and starches contain no cholesterol and little or no saturated fat. Vegetable fats usually are polyunsaturated.

HIGH BLOOD PRESSURE

Your blood pressure should be evaluated on your initial visit with your physician. You should have it monitored and reviewed on a regular basis if it is not in a normal range.

Experience has shown that in a large percentage of patients the blood pressure decreases proportionally with the decrease in weight.

Because high blood pressure is primarily related to excess weight, weight loss is usually the first recommendation to assist in regulation before any other measures are taken, including medication.

Also linked to high blood pressure is salt intake. This diet is low sodium and very low in foods containing high amounts of salt.

"Internal illness reflects external conditions."

WATER AND WEIGHT LOSS

Water is a healing and rejuvenating therapy, particularly to those who do not drink enough. The balance of body fluids depends on having a consistent supply of pure water.

One of the first steps to weight loss is to increase water intake to at least 2-3 quarts a day.

Many people think that drinking too much water will cause them to retain water. Just the opposite is true. If the body is not receiving an adequate water supply it will retain fluids at all costs. The body withholds water from the kidneys, and the urine becomes scanty and highly concentrated.

It works like this: With proper water intake, kidney function improves and many waste products are flushed out. This relieves the liver so it can metabolize the stored fats into energy. As toxins and excessive salt are flushed out, the body no longer needs to hold onto water to dilute the toxins. Thus, drinking more water relieves water retention.

Also, the bowels work better with additional water as the body does not need to extract water from the colon for its metabolic needs. Constipation is relieved. This also relieves the liver of having to deal with the bowel toxins so it can work on metabolizing fat.

With water relieving the liver, its function is improved and it is better able to humanize some of those airborne proteins (pollens), such as cedar and ragweed, that cause allergies. Many allergies are caused by the inability of the liver to disarm unusual proteins.

Studies have shown that water not only is a natural suppressant to the appetite, but helps the body metabolize stored fat. A decrease in water intake will cause fat deposits to increase, while drinking more water can actually reduce fat deposits.

Drinking your required water ensures that toxins and excessive salts will be flushed out. If you drink more than your body requires, the surplus is promptly and easily eliminated. However, do not exceed more than 1 gallon (4 quarts) per day.

The more water you drink, the more stored water and metabolized fat will be released and flushed out. People with excess weight will have larger metabolic loads and, since water is the key to fat metabolism, they need to drink more. As this increased fat metabolism is being shed, drinking more water helps flush out the system.

Another beneficial factor to water is the benefits to your skin and the cells that prevent sagging and that haggard look. As you lose weight the water that is absorbed into the skin cells actually buoys the cells.

With proper water intake, kidney function improves, more waste products are flushed out, and this in turn helps the liver to metabolize the stored fats (cellulite) into energy.

THERE IS NO SUBSTITUTION FOR WATER

With any other liquid, such as weak tea or diet colas, the kidneys still have to work to metabolize the electrolytes (sodium, potassium, and so on). The water simply allows the kidneys to work at their top efficiency and to flush the system of the fat being metabolized.

The majority of your water should be drunk throughout the day and finished prior to your last meal of the day. Try not to drink in the evening to avoid spending the night in and out of the bathroom.

WATER RETENTION

Water retention is variable from individual to individual. The amount of water you retain has nothing to do with the amount of water you drink.

If fluid intake is insufficient, the body will retain water to maintain a balance. Fat tissue holds about 15% of water whether a person is overweight or not. As you lose weight, the adipose tissue and the skin may not shrink back to the prior fat level as fast as the fat is being lost. As a result the empty space temporarily gets filled with fluid. This fluid will eventually disappear as the skin and underlying tissues shrink.

For this reason we tend to discourage diuretics, as they offer a temporary solution at best. The body will naturally correct itself if given time; you should realize this is not a setback.

SOME CAUSES OF WATER RETENTION:
Menstrual cycle (before and during)

Ovulation (during)
A hot day, sunburn
Strenuous exercise
Not drinking enough fluids
Excess salt in your diet
Certain medications

SIGNS AND SYMPTOMS:

Swollen hands (rings tight)
Swollen feet or ankles (shoes tight)
Decreased urination
Swollen eyes
General bloated feeling
Weight gain with no dietary errors

NATURAL DIURETICS AND PREVENTION SUGGESTIONS:

Drink more water
Avoid getting overheated
Adequate moderate exercise
Deep, relaxed rest

NATURAL DIURETICS:

Drink parsley tea. Boil a handful of fresh parsley in one quart of water for five minutes. Add a tea bag for about one minute.
Asparagus
Vitamin B-6 with herb tea
K-B-11 (a combination of Uva Ursi, watermelon tea, shave grass, juniper berry, corn silk, buchu leaves, and chickweed)
Any herbal diuretic

SODIUM AND WATER

Sodium (salt) helps regulate the passage of water and nutrients out of cells and helps maintain the proper acid-base balance in body fluids.

The average diet furnishes about three times as much sodium as is needed. Your diet is low sodium to decrease water retention and lower blood pressure. Because the body is two-thirds water and salt contributes to retention of body fluids, we highly recommend, especially on the program, the reduction of salt intake and foods high in salt content. Avoid refined, heated table salt. Use evaporated sea salt instead.

Eight Glasses a Day Keep the Fat Away!

Water suppresses the appetite naturally and helps the body metabolize stored fat.

Kidneys can't function properly without enough water. When they don't work to capacity, some of their load is dumped onto the liver. The liver's primary function is to metabolize stored fat into usable energy for your body. However, if the liver had to do some of the kidney's work, it can't operate to its full potential. If that happens, it will metabolize less fat, and more fat will remain stored in the body, and your weight loss will stop.

If you are retaining fluid, drinking water is the best treatment. When the body doesn't get enough water it perceives this as a threat to survival and begins to hold onto all of it. Water is stored on the outside of the cells as swollen feet, hands, and legs.

Taking a diuretic is just a temporary solution and is not recommended. If you have a high salt intake your body will tolerate only so much sodium and only in a certain concentration. The more salt you have, the more water your system will retain to dilute it. Drinking your water forces the sodium through the kidneys and flushes out excess salt.

Exercising requires more water to maintain proper muscle tone by giving muscles their natural ability to contract and by preventing dehydration.

It may also help to decrease or prevent the sagging skin that usually follows major weight loss. The shrinking cells are buoyed by water, which plumps the skin and leaves it clear, healthy, and resilient.

One of the biggest jobs the water will do during your weight loss program is to flush the body of toxins and waste. All the metabolized fat must go somewhere. As you are losing the weight, the discarded fat must get out of the body somehow and go somewhere. If it remains in you, you may become more toxic and retain or gain weight.

Headaches, stomach aches, and general crankiness can often accompany weight loss, especially in the beginning, due to all the toxins moving and being flushed out. It's a good sign—just ride it out. It doesn't last long and it is very beneficial.

How much water should you drink? During the diet, eight glasses a day are required. Even the average person should drink eight glasses every day. A person trying to lose weight should actually drink an additional glass for every 25 pounds of excess weight. If you have an intense exercise session you should increase the amount, and during the summer it is recommended that you increase your water intake.

Water should be cold. Cold water is absorbed into the system more quickly than tap water.

When you are giving the body the amount of water that it needs to function optimally, its fluids are balanced. When this happens, you reach a "breakthrough point." That means that the endocrine gland functions improve. The fluid retention is alleviated as stored water is lost, and more fat is used as fuel because the liver is free to metabolize stored fat. Natural thirst returns and a loss of hunger occurs almost overnight.

Incredible as it may seem, water is quite possibly the single most important catalyst in losing weight and maintaining the weight loss. Permanent weight loss is definitely connected to your body fluids being in balance and functioning to their maximum potential. Drinking water may be the cheapest, easiest, and healthiest way to lose weight and keep it off permanently.

A Word About Water

Volumes could be written about the importance of water. It is critical to nutrition in that it helps digest, absorb, and transport nutrients throughout the body. The chemical reactions in the body occur in a saltwater solution. Water carries colloidal minerals that are used for cellular function.

Both the rule that you should drink eight glasses a day and the fact that three quarters of the body is water should give you the message that it's just plain crucial to have enough pure water every day.

Unfortunately, most of the water on this "water planet" is now contaminated with chemicals, pesticides, radiation, bacteria, giardia, amoebas, and other pollutants. Tap water is often unfit for drinking. It is not conducive to good health. Spring waters are often contaminated too. Distilled waters are dead (the bioavailability is low due to the heat-altered shape of the molecule and its estrangement from the earth). The time has come to re-evaluate the ways that we provide for ourselves and our families to have pure, bioavailable, soft, clean, and living water.

If you have an interest in upgrading your water system for you and your family, here are a few ways that we recommend:

1.   Use a high-quality, well-maintained reverse osmosis water purification system.

2.   Use distilled water that has been enlivened with 1 teaspoon of sea water per gallon plus 10 drops of stabilized oxygen plus 6 hours of sitting in the sunlight.

3.   Use bottled waters, such as Volvic, Evian, or Perrier, when in restaurants.

LABELS

Food labels can be instrumental in helping you choose low-fat, low-calorie, healthful foods. They can also provide you with some confusing and, in some cases, misleading information.

Labeling regulations have been revised several times since the Food and Drug Administration began regulating food labels in 1906. Currently, all labels must state the following information:

Name of product; name and address of the manufacturer, packer, or distributor; net contents in terms of weight, measure, or count; list of ingredients in descending order of predominance by weight.

The exception to the ingredient-listing requirement is foods that have a "standard of identity." By that we mean that these foods have standard ingredients established by the government. Included in this list are foods such as ice cream, ketchup, pasta, and mayonnaise. Some manufacturers of these goods have listed their ingredients anyway.

The ingredient list is useful consumer information, but it still does not give the whole picture. It helps to identify saturated fats, salt, and other ingredients that you will be trying to avoid. However, specific spices, colors, and flavors don't have to be named. These will often be listed generally under "artificial flavoring," "spices," or "artificial coloring."

The order of the ingredients may also be of some help in identifying how much of certain ingredients are present, but it doesn't specify exact amounts. If a label lists flour as the first ingredient and vegetable oil as the second, this could mean that flour makes up 60 percent of the weight and oil makes up 39 percent, meaning that the product is a high-fat item. However, flour might comprise 98 percent of the weight and oil only 1 percent, making the product a low-fat item.

Specific nutritional labeling helps clarify some of this but is not required on all food labels. The FDA requires nutritional information on any food product that:

1. Has nutrients added to it, such as fortified cereal.
2. Makes a nutritional claim, such as "low in cholesterol."
3. Is prepared for special dietary uses, such as baby formula.

All other nutritional labeling is voluntary on the part of each manufacturer. Currently, about 60 percent of food products have these labels.

The labels must also contain information pertaining to nutritional claims. If the product is labeled "low cholesterol," it must specify the milligrams of cholesterol per serving. Manufacturers may also list optional information: a breakdown of fat content (amounts of saturated and polyunsaturated fat), a breakdown of carbohydrate content (simple sugars, complex carbohydrates, and fiber), fiber content by itself, or U.S. RDA percentages of other vitamins and minerals.

Besides having guidelines on what manufacturers must put on a label, the FDA also has specific regulations for what may not be stated. The following types of statements are not allowed:

A natural vitamin is better than a synthetic one.

You can't get adequate nutrients from a balanced diet consisting of regular food.

A food can be used to prevent, treat, or cure a disease.

A food has a dietary effect or quality that has no proven significance in human nutrition.

The soil in which a food is grown makes it deficient in nutrients or quality.

The storage, transportation, processing, or cooking makes a food inadequate or deficient.

These regulations do not stop manufacturers from making statements that are misleading. An example of this would be the "no cholesterol" label. The fact that there is no cholesterol in a product does not mean it contains no saturated fat. Snack crackers could be labeled "no cholesterol" even if they contain highly saturated coconut oil. Consumers who are not aware that saturated fats have a greater influence on blood cholesterol levels than dietary cholesterol would think this label claim makes the crackers a good choice.

LABEL TERMINOLOGY

Diet or Dietetic:
May be reduced in calories, sodium, or sugar.

Enriched or Fortified:
Has added vitamins, minerals, or protein.

Extra Lean (meat and poultry):
Has no more than 5 percent fat by weight.

Imitation:
Pertains to a food that is a substitute for and resembles another food, but is nutritionally inferior to that food. Nutritionally inferior means there is a reduction in the amount of an essential nutrient, but does not include a reduction in calorie or fat content.

Lean (meat and poultry):
Contains no more than 10 percent fat by weight.

Leaner (meat and poultry):
Has at least 25 percent less fat than the standard.

Low Calorie:
Contains no more than 40 calories per serving or no more than 0.4 calorie per gram.

Low Sodium:
Contains 140 mg. or less sodium per serving.

Natural:
Can mean anything, including foods containing additives; there is no clear definition as yet.

No Cholesterol:
Contains no cholesterol, but may contain saturated fats.

Organic:
Can mean anything; no regulations govern it as yet.

Reduced Calorie:
Has one-third fewer calories than the original product and must include a comparison of the original product and the reduced calorie version.

Reduced Sodium:
The usual level of sodium in a product has been reduced by at least 75 percent.

Sodium Free:
Contains less than 5 mg. sodium per serving.

Sugar-Free or Sugarless:
Contains no table sugar, but may contain any of the following, which have the same amount of calories as sugar: honey, fructose, corn syrup, or sorbitol. Products may also be high in fat and calories.

Unsalted, No Salt Added, or Without Added Salt:
No salt has been added in processing, but the food may still contain other sodium-containing ingredients.

Very Low Sodium:
Has 35 mg. or less per serving.

Even knowing the terminology doesn't always clarify the nutritional value. The name of a product often contains a meaning that consumers are unaware of and may be very misleading. In the case of processed foods with meat or poultry, the government has regulations on names of the product. "Beef with macaroni" must have more beef than macaroni, while "macaroni with beef" has more macaroni than beef.

Another misleading and confusing product label is that of juices. Here is a list that might assist you in your selections (especially for children):

Fruit Juice: 100 percent real fruit juice

Drink:
Contains 35-69 percent real fruit juice.

Fruit Drink:
Has 10-34 percent juice.

Fruit-Flavored Drink:
Contains 10 percent or less fruit juice or no juice at all.

Light is something on the inside too.

Label Update

Soon to be gone are the food packages claiming to serve 2-3/4 servings. Terms such as *fresh*, *light*, and *natural* will no longer be misleading. By spring of 1994 nearly all food packages will display nutritional labels that adhere to the new regulations established by the FDA. All retailers have until July 1994 to comply with the regulations; you will begin to see the labels soon.

Research has linked foods to certain health benefits or health risks, so it just makes good sense to read labels and learn to understand their meaning before you purchase and make your food choices.

The nutrition fact labels found on foods will have to display more complete, accurate, and easy-to-understand information. Under the *new* guidelines, you'll find the following information on most food labels:

Serving Size: For the first time, serving sizes for all similar foods must be consistent. Consistent serving sizes make it easier for you to compare nutritional values.

Calories and calories from fat: Along with the number of calories per serving, the labels must include the number of calories coming from fat. This number will help you limit your fat intake to less than 30 percent of total caloric intake, which is the recommended level.

Daily Values for nutrients: The all-new "Daily Values" section of the label will show you how a food fits into the overall daily diet. Given as percentages, the daily values will tell the food's nutritional content based on a 2,000-calorie daily diet because it has the greatest health benefits.

According to the American Dietetic Association, children younger than age 11 and older adults should refer to the 2,000-calorie diet as a guide. The 2,500-calorie range should serve as a guide for men, pregnant women, and children older than age 11. Remember that these are only guides and each person's needs will vary.

Calories per gram: The bottom section of the label will show you how many calories are in each gram of fat, carbohydrate, and protein.

There are special exceptions under which some foods will not have Nutrition Facts (NF). These include:

Foods produced by a small business or foods produced and sold on site (bakeries), vending machine foods, foods shipped in bulk such as flour shipped to cafeterias, coffee, tea, and some spices.

Fresh fruits and vegetables, raw poultry, meat, and fish. The NF are voluntary for many raw foods, but retailers will be strongly advised by the FDA to display this information for the most frequently eaten fruits, vegetables, and fish.

Packages that are too small to display the information. Instead, the manufacturers must include a phone number or address that consumers can call or write for the information.

The USDA, which regulates meat and poultry, has issued regulations requiring nutritional labeling on processed meat and poultry products. Labeling for fresh meat and poultry will be voluntary.

Once-ambiguous label terms, such as *light* or *less*, now have meaningful definitions. Below are some of what the most common terms will mean:

Reduced, Less, or Fewer: A food that has been nutritionally changed or reformulated to contain at least 25 percent fewer calories than the regular or reference food. For example, a *reduced fat* cheesecake must contain 25 percent less fat than regular cheesecake, or pretzels may claim to have 25 percent *less fat* than potato chips.

Free: Any product containing very small or insignificant amounts of fat, saturated fat, cholesterol, sodium or salt, sugars, or calories. For example, *calorie free* means fewer than 5 calories per serving. *Sugar free* or *fat free* both mean the food has less than 0.5 gram of sugar or fat per serving. *Without, no,* and *zero* are also approved terms that can be used in place of *free*.

Low: Used on foods that may be eaten daily in reasonable amounts without exceeding the dietary guidelines for fat, cholesterol, sodium, or calories. The term may be used in these ways:
    Low fat: 3 grams or less per serving
    Low saturated fat: 1 gram or less per serving and not more than 15 percent of calories from saturated fat

Low sodium: 140 mg. or less per serving
Very low sodium: 35 mg. or less per serving
Low cholesterol: 20 mg. or less per serving
Low calorie: 40 calories or less per serving
Little, few, and *low source of* may also be used instead of low.

High: A food containing 20 percent or more of the daily value for a desirable nutrient (such as vitamin C) per serving. *Rich in* or *excellent source* may also be used instead of *high.*

Good Source: Reserved for foods that contain 10-19 percent of the daily value per serving for a specific nutrient, such as fiber or calcium. Alternate terms are *contains* or *provides.*

Light or lite: There is more than one approved definition for the term *light* or lite. When describing a product that contains at least one-third fewer calories or 50 percent less fat than the reference food, the term *light* or *lite* may be used. Or the term may be used if the sodium content of a low-calorie, low-fat product has been reduced by 50 percent. For example, if *light* is listed on the label of a cottage cheese product, it may refer to any of these definitions. However, the one that applies must be specified on the label —such as *light in fat.* Light may still be used to describe texture or color if the label explains this reference.

More: This term may describe any food containing at least 10 percent more of the daily value for protein, vitamins, minerals, dietary fiber, or potassium than the reference food. For example, an iron-rich bread may claim to contain *more iron* than the reference bread.

Lean and extra lean: These may refer only to the fat content of meats, poultry, seafood, or game meats. *Lean*: less than 10 grams fat, less than 4 grams saturated fat, and less than 95 mg. cholesterol per serving and per 100 grams of the product's weight. *Extra lean:* less than 5 grams fat, less than 2 grams saturated fat, and less than 95 mg. cholesterol per serving and per 100 grams of the product's weight.

Fresh: Used only to describe a raw or unprocessed food that has never been frozen, heated, or preserved. *Fresh frozen, frozen fresh,* and *freshly frozen* are allowed on foods that have been quickly frozen while fresh. Certain foods, such as milk and bread, are exempt from this regulation if the food is generally accepted by consumers as fresh.

VITAMINS AND MINERALS

Vitamins are essential for chemical reactions throughout the body. Our bodies cannot manufacture most vitamins, so they need to be provided in the foods we eat. However, the world is changing and many of our old philosophies must change also. A hundred years ago, you would not have needed a supplement. All the vitamins and minerals you needed would have come from proper diet. The earth bountifully supported human nutrition.

Today, you're not going to get what you need to cope with the chemically toxic air, chemically treated water, radiation in our atmosphere, the inadvertent chemically treated and pesticide-poisoned foods, deficient ozone layer, and the stresses of our fast-paced lifestyles. You're certainly not going to get it from foods grown in depleted soil with chemical fertilizers, hybridized for shelf life, picked green, stored, artificially ripened, and transported for days to your supermarket.

While it's true that all the vitamins you need in a year could be held in a thimble, and that too much supplementation is detrimental, people must supplement with low-potency, natural supplements to ensure that the 46 essential nutrients the body must have are provided.

"Essential" nutrients must come from food—20 minerals, 15 vitamins, 9 amino acids, and 2 fatty acids.

To be deficient is synonymous with degeneration. It is estimated that 90 percent of the population is deficient in an essential nutrient. To have optimal health you must have all 46 essential nutrients.

Therefore, we require you to take a vitamin-mineral supplement of your choice daily. Supplement wisely with a low-potency, natural, sugarless, herb-based formula. Take your supplement with a specific meal (breakfast) to create habit and to prevent an upset stomach (especially if it's high in iron).

Women should consider taking a supplement that also contains added iron and calcium. Sources of calcium and iron in foods are tofu, skim milk, low-fat cottage cheese, collard and turnip greens, fresh herring, broccoli, and kale. Specific sources of iron are lean meat, fish, poultry, enriched breads and cereals, liver, shrimp, and leafy green vegetables.

Vitamins and minerals perform specific functions, most often with an enzyme. They have no useful metabolic function by themselves. The body has a maximum limit of production for each enzyme, so only the approximate amount established by the RDA for a vitamin or mineral can combine with the nutrient's corresponding enzyme.

Increasing vitamins or minerals will not stimulate a greater production of the enzyme or an increase in your metabolic function, such as immunity or utilization of fat stores. Actually, the body will increase urinary excretion of the unused nutrient if the nutrient is water soluble. Too much can cause a build-up to toxic levels or even interfere with the absorption or metabolism of other nutrients.

It is difficult to establish general guidelines on the maximum safety limit for each vitamin or mineral. Consume no more than three times the U.S. RDA for any vitamin or mineral.

The word *natural* on the label sounds great but it does little more than increase the cost. Vitamins do not exist naturally apart from food. They are either synthesized in the laboratory or extracted from food through a process that exposes them to chemical solvents. Minerals, however, are natural since they are fundamental elements that cannot be synthesized.

The word organic is used carelessly also. Unless it is grown on selenium- or chromium-rich soil that incorporates the minerals into its structure in an organic form, it does nothing more than increase the cost too.

Chelation minerals are chemically bound to another substance, usually an amino acid, that can be naturally occurring or synthetic. Supposedly, this improves the absorption and utilization of a mineral. The chelation forms a weak bond between the mineral and the amino acid but the bond is easily broken once the supplement reaches your stomach. The benefits of chelation are more theory than fact at this time. The only benefit of chelation is that these minerals, such as zinc gluconate, are less irritating to your stomach and intestine than are the mineral salts, such as zinc sulfate.

The "time-released" supplements are a single large dose of a vitamin or mineral that causes blood levels of the nutrient to rise abruptly, which stimulates the kidneys to excrete the excess nutrient. Time-released supplements are intended to dissolve slowly in the intestine.

However, most require 6 hours to disintegrate and studies show only about 14% of the supplement is absorbed. Most of the time-released supplement is excreted unchanged in the stool.

The very best source of nutrients is your food. The optimal levels of all vitamins and minerals cannot be guaranteed on any diet that contains less than 1,600-2,000 calories a day. That is why it is recommended that you choose a vitamin-mineral supplement that provides a safe and cost-effective "insurance" that the daily nutrient needs are met at a time when you are establishing new eating habits for a lifetime of health.

If you have any medical conditions, you should always obtain approval from your physician or dietitian before initiating a supplement program.

The chief cause for going off a diet
is trading what we want the "most"
for what we want in the "moment."

SNACKS

Snacks as a rule are not advisable. The body is resting in between its digestive duties and preparing enzymes for your next meal.

If you find it necessary to snack, make sure that it is done at least 3 hours after lunch.

SOME SUGGESTIONS ABOUT SNACKING

First of all, the desire for snacks will disappear gradually as your well-nourished body's blood sugar stabilizes, stamina and steadfast energy become natural, and the sugar-craving symptoms will usually be gone within 2-4 weeks.

If you do have strong sugar cravings, it may be due to protein deficiency at a cellular level so, as you build your protein base, you will be gradually eliminating the need for sugar snacks.

Do not eat proteins as a snack; they deplete the body's digestive abilities. Celery, carrot sticks, or any type of raw vegetable is always a good snack.

Design a low-calorie dip and use a vegetable platter as the mid-afternoon or dinner substitute.

Popcorn (cooked by hot air rather than in oil) is a good snack.

Fruit makes a great snack item, especially in place of that mid-afternoon or evening meal: fruit salads, frozen red grapes, seasonal fruit kabobs with nondairy Cool Whip.

Be creative and enjoy choosing and preparing these wonderful foods. Always choose fresh fruits and be sure to wash or scrub them thoroughly.

No dried, canned, or syrup-packed fruit is permitted.

Some suggestions: sugar-free popsicles (Crystal Light), Dezerta gelatin or Jell-O sugar-free gelatin, Jell-O sugar-free puddings, Ortega taco sauce or a salsa with homemade chips (pita bread cut up and warmed in the oven).

The amount of any snack should be kept to a minimum. Trust yourself and be responsible for deciding how much and when, is the general rule. A good guideline would be one cup of whatever you are eating, depending on the item and the circumstances.

GOOD ADVICE: It is important to minimize detrimental foods and maximize beneficial ones. Although this list is captioned "Strive to Avoid," the truly best advice is "Throw Away!"

STRIVE TO AVOID:

1. Highly processed foods such as sugar, white bread, noodles, cookies, crackers, and TV dinners.

2. Foods that contain chemical preservatives, dyes, and artificial flavors.

3. "Foodless" snacks. Plan for proper balance.

4. Commercial meat that has stilbestrol (DES) or other chemicals or from animals that have been inhumanely raised.

5. Fruits and vegetables that have been sprayed, fumigated, dyed, or waxed.

6. Canned fruits and vegetables—most fruits are oversweetened and many vegetables are overcooked.

7. Eggs produced by hens in small cages, force fattened, or treated with chemicals. Use fertile yard eggs instead.

8. Commercial white bread or other bakery products.

9. Hydrogenated shortenings, heat-treated oils and margarine.

10. Deep-fat frying as fatty acids break down at high temperatures. Avoid fried foods.

11. Chocolate, as it interferes with mineral assimilation and is highly allergenic and addictive to some people.

12.   Commercial milk and milk products that contain artificial coloring, flavoring, emulsifiers, sweeteners, and ice cream.

13.   Processed cow's milk: pasteurized, homogenized, dried, canned.

14.   Soft drinks with or without sugar. Avoid stimulating drinks, which exhaust the adrenal glands and the pancreas.

15.   Coffee. Use water-processed decaf in transition. Pekoe teas (black teas) also have caffeine.

16.   Sugar (in all its many forms), synthetic sweeteners.

17.   Any product with preservatives, BHA, BHT, nitrates, nitrites, sodium bisulfide.

18.   Commercial peanut butter.

19.   Commercial cooking oils (hydrogenated). Use an extra-virgin olive oil. Refrigerate after opening.

20.   Sulfured, dried fruit.

21.   Refined, heated table salt. Use evaporated sea salt.

22.   Salted, roasted nuts.

SOME BASIC SUGGESTIONS:

1.   Cook only in stainless steel, Corning or enamel ware, or glass. Do not use aluminum or pressure cookers.
2.   Use butter instead of substitutes. For a spread high in unsaturated fats, blend 1/2 lb. sweet cream butter and 1/2 cup sesame oil. Add a little lecithin and vitamin E.
3.   Use pure drinking water liberally. Avoid tap water.
4.   Use soups often.
5.   Use a natural sea salt sparingly.
6.   Use a variety of herbs and spices in cooking—parsley, basil, thyme, rosemary, sage, nutmeg, cinnamon, dill—for food interest and for stimulating the appetite and the gastric juices.
7.   Use vinegars occasionally to maintain good gastric acidity. They do wonders for soups.

A SUCCESSFUL JOURNEY

Diets are full of challenges! But then, you already know that. The key to supporting your diet is long-range planning. Always keep your goals in sight, even if you fall off the diet. Get right back on and keep your end result in mind.

PLAN YOUR MEALS IN ADVANCE
Sit down at the table. Use utensils, take small portions, and then take more if you're still hungry. It's impossible to think up properly balanced and limited-calorie meals on the spur of the moment.

EAT SLOWLY
Stay within the body's speed limit. This allows the brain time to register the food you eat and stop the impulses that make you think you're hungry. By eating too fast you override the brain-to-stomach circuitry that tells you to quit. You become full, then overfull, before the brain can turn off the desire to eat.

EAT CONSCIOUSLY
Be aware of the food you're eating. Taste it, touch the texture, smell it, feel temperature. Don't try to eat when you're in the middle of a conversation. Stay focused on your food and savor!

CHEW YOUR FOOD
Set your fork or spoon down between bites, chew slowly, take your time, acknowledge what had to happen for that particular food item to get to your table.

STAY OUT OF THE KITCHEN
Do not cruise the kitchen out of habit, or scan the refrigerator. Don't spend the whole day baking.

ASK FOR SUPPORT
Learn to receive support, to accept it graciously. Enlist your friends and family to support you. Let them know how important this is for you. Ask them not to undermine what you're trying to do for yourself. If they aren't willing to assist, avoid them until you have reached your goals.

THINK THIN

Use positive reminders. Put a picture of a slender person on the refrigerator that has the image that you would like to emulate. Have a very clear image of what that slender "new you" will look and feel like. Begin acting as if you are that slender person *now*! Have this image so well defined that you know exactly how you will feel emotionally, physically, and mentally.

'If all you do is worry
about what could have been,
or fear what might be,
you will never know what is here now.'

DEBBIE

When Debbie first started I could tell that she was very sceptical. I asked why she felt that we couldn't help her. She told me that she had been to Nutri-System, Jenny Craig, Diet-Center and Weight Watchers and had failed to lose any significant weight.

She had set twenty five pounds as her goal weight. She did relate to me that she was very relived when she discovered that we had no high pressure sales people and their were no contracts involved. I explained that our clinic was run like any other medical doctors office and if for any reason she was not completely satisfied she could discontinue without any one making her feel guilty or that she had failed.

Still a little skeptical, she had her physical and started the program that day. About ten days later she came into my office and told me that she couldn't believe it. She had lost seven pounds. I didn't see her for another three weeks, and she seemed delighted to tell me that she had lost a total of thirteen pounds.

She lost the rest in an additional four weeks and reached her goal. Since that time she has referred literally dozen of friends and co-workers to our clinic and I consider Debbie one of our real success stories.

THE PATH WITH A HEART

Anything is one of a million paths. Therefore you must always keep in mind that a path is only a path. If you feel you should not follow it, you must not stay with it under any conditions. To have such clarity you must lead a disciplined life. Only then will you know that any path is only a path, and there is no affront, to oneself or to others, in dropping it if that is what your heart tells you to do. But your decision to keep on the path or to leave it must be free of fear or ambition.

I warn you. Look at every path closely and deliberately. Try it as many times as you think necessary. Then ask yourself, and yourself alone, one question. This question is one that only a very old man asks. My benefactor told me about it once when I was young, and my blood was too vigorous for me to understand it. Now I do understand it. I will tell you what it is: Does this path have a heart?

All paths are the same: they lead nowhere. They are paths going through the bush or into the bush. In my own life I could say I have traversed long, long paths, but I am not anywhere. My benefactor's question has meaning now. Does this path have a heart? If it does, the path is good; if it doesn't, it is of no use.

Both paths lead nowhere; but one has a heart, the other doesn't. One makes for a joyful journey; as long as you follow it, you are one with it. The other will make you curse your life. One makes you strong; the other weakens you.

The trouble is that nobody asks the question; and when a man finally realizes that he has taken a path without a heart, the path is ready to kill him. At that point very few men can stop to deliberate, and leave the path.

A path without heart is never enjoyable. You have to work hard even to take it. On the other hand, a path with heart is easy; it does not make you work at liking it.

For me there is only the traveling on paths that have heart, on any path that may have heart. There I travel, and the only worthwhile challenge is to traverse its full length. And there I travel looking, looking, breathlessly.

—Don Juan, a Yaqui warrior; as told to Carlos Castaneda

CHAPTER EIGHT

Out Post

POST-PROGRAM ALTERNATIVES

This section of the book is for those of you who have an additional interest in furthering your knowledge about foods, nutrition, preventative techniques, and wellness suggestions after you finish your weight loss program.

The intention of this material is to offer an extension of information for lifetime maintenance, information that may assist you in forming your own permanent and personal maintenance lifestyle and ideals. However, this material is *not* required for your weight loss program.

This information is here to further assist you in some basic alternatives about your body and some of its functions. Continuing your education about your health is a decision that only you can make. This information goes beyond the program in order for you to implement some of its guidelines into your lifestyle if you choose to do so.

At the back of this book you will find additional recommendations and suggested reading in many of the areas that are covered.

This section is not meant to dictate use of any technique as a form of treatment for specific medical problems without the advice of your own physician. The intent of this material is only to offer information of a general nature to help you cooperate with your doctor in your mutual quest for health and wellness and a natural sense of well-being.

"There is a place within you
where you know your own answers,
that part of you
that is pure love and all knowing."

PROTEINS

PROTEINS: THE MAIN BODY BUILDER

Protein is necessary to build, maintain, and repair the body. It also helps produce antibodies that support warding off disease, and enzymes and hormones that regulate many of our body processes.

With so many purposes, protein is quickly used in the body. Adults require about 65 grams of protein daily. Protein is made up of 22 components called amino acids. Fourteen of the amino acids can be manufactured by the body if they aren't found in the food that is consumed. However, the remaining eight amino acids must be supplied by the food that is eaten. All eight of the essential amino acids should be eaten at the same meal for the protein to be properly used by the body.

Proteins take longer to metabolize but provide a sustained energy matrix within which the carbohydrates in transit in the body fluids can operate without spiking and creating deficits. When protein and carbohydrates are eaten together the body has to choose one; it cannot break down and digest both. The carbohydrate almost always loses. It goes into the body to become stored and begins to putrefy.

Optimal use of proteins would be to eat them as early in the day as possible (5 a.m. until 3 p.m). Proteins eaten early assist in the acid and alkaline swing, provide sustained energy during the day, signal the release of amino acids and nutrients, build tissue integrity, and provide the body's best digestive powers. Proteins eaten later in the day interfere with sleep, are not properly digested or metabolized, disrupt the cleansing and detoxifying mode, disturb the regenerative alkaline sleep cycle, sit in the lymphatic system all night and contribute to congestion, and become toxic.

Eat proteins with vegetables. Raw vegetables provide enzymes that assist in digesting proteins, whereas lightly cooked vegetables provide inner cell factors rich in DNA and RNA, the building blocks of body revitalization.

Eat proteins with a small amount of oil. Before a protein can be used by the body, it must be made nontoxic by the liver.

Eat proteins away from carbohydrates. If protein is eaten at the same time as a carbohydrate, digestion is compromised, the body becomes a breeding ground for bacteria, and cholesterol levels run high.

Eat proteins without sugars (refined carbohydrates). They give a quick energy rush, excite the system, and then drop the energy level off quickly, leaving an energy deficit.

Eat proteins in small portions. Larger volumes result in waste and toxins from fermentation. Smaller portions create better nutrition and more energy.

Try not to drink liquids with proteins; they may dilute the hydrochloric acid needed to digest proteins.

Eat as much of the low-stress proteins as possible.

Eat proteins as meals, not as snacks. Snacks deplete the body's digestive abilities and increase the chances for putrefaction.

Eat proteins without fruits. Fruits are actually in a class to be eaten alone.

If the liver is healthy it can convert the essential amino acids into most of what the body needs. If the liver is toxic, swollen, sluggish, or congested, you need to supply it with complete amino acids so that it can cleanse and repair itself as well as perform its other duties. It's not always what we eat that nourishes the body. . . it could be what the liver processes!

Unfamiliar to most weight loss diets being touted today is toxicity control, yet toxicity can be a primary cause of excessive weight, particularly in those who have problems losing weight and keeping it off. Other factors can include an underactive or overactive pituitary or thyroid gland and excessive caloric intake (overeating high-calorie foods), but a major consideration is toxicity.

When the liver is congested and overburdened in its role as a blood detoxifier, the body surrounds toxic debris with a mantle of fat and increases water retention to keep it from harming the organs and tissues. When a person diets (fasts or reduces calories) to lose weight, the fat is metabolized and weight is lost, but often the toxins are not removed because nothing was done about the liver. Instead they stay suspended in the bloodstream and lymphatic system because the liver is congested and is not able to detoxify the body as soon as the person eats again, even if it is just a small meal, and the weight is piled back on again.

It is not uncommon to hear of a person who loses 12 pounds, eats a 14-oz. meal, and gains 12 pounds back again. After suffering the trauma of a weight reduction diet, the weight magically reappears and the final insult is that in cases the weight gain is greater than what was originally lost!

This often happens to those who attempt the "protein powder skip a meal" program. Along with the reduction in calories, it is important for most people to release the retained toxins. An overactive appestat (hypothalamus) center in the brain, which encourages a person to eat and sends out the signal that a person is hungry, responds well to nutrition specific to the pituitary and hypothalamus.

A sugar craving (hypoglycemic reaction) is generally triggered by an insufficient amount of usable protein in the body, particularly at the cellular level. Note: There may be too much protein in the diet, but it's not being digested and handled by the liver.

Nutrition that enhances the assimilation of amino acids in the tissues, as well as proper preparation of proteins, is indicated. Few people realize that hypoglycemia is much more a liver issue than a pancreatic problem. It's the liver that sets the glucose (sugar) level of the blood. The pancreas only provides the insulin to introduce the glucose to the cells. Sugar cravings can also be a lack of B vitamins. If a high dose of B vitamins is applied, the lack is met, but then the B vitamins can stimulate the craving for food.

For weight reduction, it is recommended to use a gentle potency B-complex as well as a mega-vitamin. Colon support is always recommended for weight loss programs, as is kidney support. This enhances the elimination process. Increase water consumption!

It is important to supply more than one source of protein. Select from a variety of the proteins available in order to provide a greater nutritional value. A variety of protein sources has the advantage of synergism and wholeness.

When protein structures are readily available, the liver doesn't have to work as hard. Just because the body is willing to compensate doesn't mean we should make it do so. The liver's job is organizing and restructuring proteins. If it is well supplied with an assortment of proteins, its ability to do its job will be enhanced.

'The word **protein** *is derived from the Greek language and means 'of primary importance.''*

CARBOHYDRATES

CARBOHYDRATES: THE BODY'S ENERGY SOURCE

Carbohydrates are another source of energy, but generally are lower in calories than are fats. They free protein for other uses and are important carriers of vitamins and minerals.

They are available in two basic forms: sugars and starches. They exist as natural sugars in fresh fruits, vegetables, and some dairy products. The only nutritional contribution sugar itself (both natural and refined) can make to your diet is calories for energy. The calorie content of foods high in refined sugars far outweighs the nutrient value; on the other hand, foods such as fruits supply you with not only the energy but also the essential nutrients.

If you restrict the carbohydrate intake, your body will simply compensate by manufacturing energy from protein, creating a nutritional deficit. The trade-off of using valuable protein instead of carbohydrates for energy isn't worth the cost and will ultimately lead to poor nutrition.

On the scale, the individual may actually be the normal weight for height but still does not feel like his or her natural weight. A full-length look at your nude body will disclose that some areas still have their deposits.

The reason for this is as follows: When an obese person reduces by starvation, type 1 and type 2 fats are always burned first because they are kept in a "current account" and are more readily available. Then, when these become exhausted, the obese person will begin to burn up the more fixed, abnormal reserves of type 3 fat. By that time, however, because of the loss of type 1 and 2 fat, the person's face may look haggard and the skin loose (where normal deposits were).

The person might feel famished, tired, weak, and hungry and usually by this time will abandon any diet. He or she may complain that you have lost in the wrong places, which is a good observation. It is this most frustrating and depressing experience that most diets can't correct.

If you have had trouble sleeping, late protein eating could be the cause. Carbohydrates tranquilize the brain through the release of sleep in an oxygen-deficient state. Complex carbohydrates take longer to metabolize and don't leave as great an energy deficit. Don't eat proteins with afternoon or evening meals. Again, combining carbohydrate with protein produces mucoid matter and insoluble cholesterols.

Many sinus and allergy symptoms are connected with eating protein and carbohydrates together. It ruins your digestion and assimilation process and creates putrefactive toxins.

The body's entire makeup is only approximately 6-12 percent carbohydrate, and most of that is in transit for energy.

High-carbohydrate diets avoid the toxicity problem of high-protein diets, but they are not in accord with the human tissue matrix and the human energy matrix. A steady stream of carbohydrates causes weak tissue and provides only superficial energy that can leave you with poor tissue integrity but cannot build strong tissue in the long run. The only people who need higher levels of carbohydrates are children and athletes. But even they must eat their carbohydrates after a proper protein matrix is provided.

Separating proteins and carbohydrates is basic food combining as taught by many leading nutritionists—that the digestion of protein and the digestion of carbohydrates are physiologically separate and conflicting functions. When carbohydrates (starches) are eaten, the digestive system sends forth alkaline or neutral gastric juices. If both of these foods are eaten together, the gastric juices (if both are provided) cancel each other out, resulting in poor digestion.

Also, since protein digestive enzymes are much more costly to the body to manufacture, if both are eaten, the body may respond only to the carbohydrate (the easier of the two digestive processes) and let the protein pass through. This results in poor absorption of amino acids and poisoning of the body due to the fermenting/decaying protein (i.e., rotten meat in the intestine).

This subject is covered in great detail by the many food-combining books available at health food stores.

VEGETABLES

Good nutrition requires both raw and lightly cooked vegetables. Here are a few guidelines with vegetables.

Of the entire amount consumed, 60% should be raw and 40% should be *lightly* cooked. The average serving should be about 1 cup.

The raw vegetables provide enzymes that help digest proteins and supply roughage to disperse proteins. *Always* eat vegetables with your protein meals.

Raw vegetables also provide protection from acids. Buffering your proteins with vegetables prevents an immune system response to the proteins and saves wear and tear on the immune system's lymphocytes.

Starchy vegetables should be minimized and nonstarchy vegetables maximized.

Raw veggies function as an escort service for improved assimilation and provide valuable minerals. Someone who has tried to eat only raw fruits and vegetables for a diet often experiences temporary improved health as they detoxify and purify the blood and lymph systems. However, eventually they waste away from inside the cells. The electrostatic charge in the inner cell diminishes in the absence of renewed chromatin factors (RNA, DNA), amino acids, and colloidal mineral factors. The ability of the cell to attract or accept nutrients is compromised.

Lightly cooked vegetables provide inner cell factors rich in DNA and RNA. Lightly cooked means quick steamed or quickly stir-fried (Chinese style). Waterless cooking, steaming, or gentle stir-frying allows the indigestible cellulose sack that surrounds the cell nucleus to break down, and your body can then absorb the DNA/RNA factors.

Do not exceed 190 degrees in your cooking, or the enzymes will begin to die. A small portion of vegetables cooked at low temperature will give the best results. Overcooked they are useless. They become acid forming, lose their ability to provide an alkaline reserve, and lose their ability to heal.

FIBER

The importance of fiber in our daily diet has been well established for years. Fiber is the part of foods that our digestive systems cannot digest and absorb, such as cellulose, pectin, and gums.

It's one of the components that makes up all plant foods (vegetables, seaweeds, fruits). Fibers in foods such as vegetables, seeds, and fruits are the very best. Tomatoes and strawberries rank at the top.

Fiber assists in the time that it takes for the food to go through the intestines. It lowers absorption of cholesterols, slows down sugar absorption, absorbs toxins and poisons for their removal from your body, adds bulk, helps to soften the stool, and is a natural preventive of constipation. It helps reduce cholesterol and triglyceride levels.

Wheat bran is not a great fiber. Its phytic acid can deplete mineral absorption by binding the minerals so they're not absorbed. It can also cause rapid introduction of sugars into the system, constipation, and gas.

However, if you feel that you should supplement fiber, flax seeds are a good source of fiber as well as of protein and oil.

FATS

Oils are fats, or lipids, that are composed of fatty acids, known as vitamin F, an essential nutrient. Vitamin F is vitally important to the thyroid and adrenal glands, nerve sheath, hair, skin, and mucous membranes. It also assists in balanced cholesterol, blood clotting, glandular function, blood pressure, and arterial flexibility.

Oils are a valuable nutrient. But misused, rancid oils are the most potentially dangerous of the food substances. Good-quality oil is essential with this diet. However, since oils are processed with different digestive enzymes than proteins, only a very small amount should be used.

The body's oil nutrient requirement is 1-2 tablespoons a day. Most can come from inside seeds and vegetables. Most of us abuse oils by frying or overheating. The hydrogenation and processing of oils turns them into poisons for our body.

Natural sources of vitamin F include raw or soaked nuts, whole grains, beans, avocado, and seeds (especially flax seed).

The real factor with regard to oils is the rancidity factor. Rancid oils as found in fried foods, cause "free radicals" that damage cells and encourage abnormal cell growth. Some foods that contain rancid oils are brown rice, chicken skin, crackers, fried foods (such as corn chips, donuts, dumplings, french fries, fried pies, and potato chips) tortilla chips, mayonnaise, nuts (roasted), rice (unless fresh, hulled) tempura, and whole-wheat products.

Here are some helpful tips on fats:

1. Grapeseed oil and sesame oil (unrefined) are best for salad because of anti-rancid factors.

2. Extra-virgin olive oil, rich in oleic acid, offers assistance t the heart by reducing the low-density lipoprotein (bad cho lesterol), while leaving the high-density lipoproteins (goo cholesterol).

3. Use sesame oil with other oils. It may prevent rancidity insid the body.

4. Learn to read labels on everything you buy so that you ca start to educate yourself about the real oil/fat ingredients i the products you buy.

5. Use grapeseed or peanut oil for cooking. It has a high flas point and doesn't get toxic as quickly as other oils.

6. Don't save or reuse heated oil.

7. When stir-frying, heat the skillet or wok to a low temperatur first and then add the oil.

8. Green olive oil is recommended once a week.

9. Store oils in refrigerator in dark-colored bottles.

10. Don't expose to warmth or light.

11. Don't shake the bottle. It contributes to oxidation.

12. Don't buy or cook fried foods.

13. Avoid wheat germ oil pearls, seed meals, lecithin (granular), commercial wheat germ, cottonseed oil, margarine, lard, shortening, commercial oils, coconut oil, palm oil, soy oil, linseed oils.

14. Use real, natural vitamin E from 100 percent vegetable sources when using oil.

15. Basmati rice, which is white in color, is superior in nutrition, low in rancid oils, and a good complex carbohydrate food.

16. Alternatives are canola, safflower, and some of the new high-oleic sunflower oils.

17. Pan fry at low temperatures. Put 2 tablespoons of water in and then add a little oil. Add your fish or vegetable mix. Cook about 3 minutes.

18. Let butter get soft at room temperature and add 1/2 cup flax seed oil. Mix and let harden in refrigerator.

19. Fresh fish and flax seed oils are richest in omega 3 oil sources. (Spectrum puts out a flax seed oil that is the richest omega-3 oil source.)

20. The best advice is to use oil sparingly, avoid rancid oils, and begin using only those oils that have been mentioned.

21. Use unsweetened, unsalted whipped butter. Fats are storage houses for your energy.

When glycogen levels are low in the liver, the body will convert the carbohydrates to fat to put an energy reserve in the bank and save it for later. Fats are energy rich, metabolize slowly, and give up energy grudgingly. Despite all the negative attitudes about fats, they are in fact essential for your good health and are a necessary part of a well-balanced food intake. Additionally, fats enable your body to use the fat-soluble vitamins, A, E, and K. They are also natural insulators and provide indispensable fatty acids that are necessary to life.

FAT REDUCTION

Probably nothing you can do for yourself would have a greater impact on your health and weight than to reduce dietary intake of the fat in your daily diet. Fat is the most concentrated source of calories, supplying more than twice—and possibly almost three times—the calories per ounce of protein or carbohydrate. Fat supplies no vitamins or minerals to compensate for its caloric density. Eating a diet high in fat is associated with elevated blood fat and cholesterol levels and increased risk for heart disease. Fat could even stimulate your appetite, decrease your body's efficiency at removing fat from storage, and encourage your weight gain, especially the solid, saturated fat.

The lower the fat content in your diet, the more foods rich in vitamins, minerals, and fiber can be included in the daily fare and the less likely you are to develop marginal nutrient deficiencies, disease, or weight problems. The calories lost when fat is removed can be replaced with nutrient-dense foods, such as whole grain breads and cereals, fruits and vegetables, and cooked dried beans and peas.

All types of fat, except the fat in saltwater fish, are strongly linked to the development of the major degenerative diseases, whereas a reduction in your fat intake reduces your risk.

Diet plays an important role in the prevention or progression of disease. A diet planned around minimally processed foods of plant origin—with limited use of lean meat, chicken, fish, low-fat or nonfat dairy products, and avoidance of added fats, salt, and sugar—reduces your risk for developing cardiovascular disease, cancer, diabetes, hypertension, and other degenerative disorders and aids in the maintenance of desired body weight.

Food labels can be particularly confusing because even a product that isn't cholesterol rich can have cholesterol buildup in your body if the fats are highly saturated. "No cholesterol" does not mean "no fat"—and that fat could be highly saturated. Read the label's nutritional content and pick foods with the highest ratio of polyunsaturated to saturated fat. The polyunsaturated fat helps the body get rid of cholesterol.

Covert Bailey's books are the very best on the market regarding fat and the diet. His books and videos are not only full of great knowledge, but they are funny and entertaining as well.

Sources of Fats and Cholesterol

Products from animal sources now provide about 58 percent of the total fat and 75 percent of the saturated fat available in the diet. Primary animal sources of fat include red meats, poultry, and fish; milk and milk products; and eggs.

Fat from vegetable sources has increased in recent years, now accounting for about 42 percent of fat available in the diet. Vegetable fat is consumed mostly in the form of plant oils such as soybean, corn, sunflower, safflower, canola, cottonseed, palm, and coconut.

In addition to direct consumption of meat products, fat is consumed in fried foods and other products, such as butter, margarine, dairy products, cheese, nuts, baked goods, salad oils, shortenings, mayonnaise, salad dressings, frostings, gravies, and sauces.

Fat is an important ingredient in many foods because of its functional properties. In many recipes, fat enhances the taste, aroma, and texture of the food. Because it is digested more slowly than protein or carbohydrates, it also plays an important role in satiety, providing a sense of fullness after eating.

Saturated fatty acids are more stable than unsaturated fatty acids because of their chemical structure. Stability is important in a cooking oil to prevent rancidity and off flavors or odors.

Dietary cholesterol is found only in animal foods. Abundant in organ meats and egg yolks, cholesterol is also contained in red meats, chicken and shellfish. Vegetable oils and shortenings are cholesterol free.

Actually, most of the cholesterol in the blood is manufactured by the body, at a rate of about 800-1,500 mg. a day, compared with 300-450 mg. consumed daily by the average American in foods.

Hydrogenated Fats

Hydrogenation is the process of adding hydrogen molecules directly to a mono-unsaturated or polyunsaturated fatty acid.

Hydrogenation is used to convert liquid oils to a semi-solid form for greater utility. For example, vegetable oils are often hydrogenated to produce shortenings or margarines. Hydrogenation also is used to

increase the stability of a fat or oil, which is important in cooking an(
extending a product's shelf-life.

All fats, particularly polyunsaturated fats, have a tendency to brea]
down or oxidize when exposed to air. Oxidized fats impart a1
undesirable, rancid flavor and odor. By adding hydrogen molecules
the fatty acids become more stable and resistant to oxidation. Thi:
is especially important for fats used in deep-fat frying.

Hydrogenation also contributes important textural properties i1
food. The degree of hydrogenation can help influence the firmnes.
and spreadability of margarines, the flakiness of pie crust, and th
creaminess of puddings.

Today, hydrogenation plays an important role in the availability an(
texture of various margarines, shortenings, baked goods, snac]
foods, cake mixes, and a wide assortment of other foods.

Fat - The Nutrient

Like carbohydrates and protein, dietary fat is an important source c
energy for the body. Fat is the most concentrated source of energ
in the diet, providing 9 calories per gram compared with 4 calorie
per gram from either carbohydrates or protein.

Dietary fat supplies essential fatty acids, such as linoleic acid, whic]
is especially important to children for proper growth. Fat is als
required for maintenance of healthy skin, regulation of cholester(
metabolism, and as a precursor of prostaglandins, hormone-lik
substances that regulate some body processes.

Dietary fat is needed to carry fat-soluble vitamins A, D, E, and K an
to aid in their absorption from the intestine. Fat also helps the bod
use carbohydrate and protein more efficiently.

The body uses whatever fat it needs for energy, and the rest is store
in various fatty tissues. Some fat is found in blood plasma and othe
body cells, but the largest amount is stored in the body's adipose (fa
cells.

These fat deposits not only store energy, but also are important i
insulating the body and supporting and cushioning organs.

What Is Fat?

Technically, fats should be referred to in the plural, since there is no one type of fat. Fats are composed of the same three elements as carbohydrates—carbon, hydrogen, and oxygen. However, fats have relatively more carbon and hydrogen, and less oxygen, thus supplying the higher fuel value of 9 calories per gram.

One molecule of a fat can be broken down into three molecules of fatty acids and one of glycerol. Thus, fats are known chemically as triglycerides.

Fats are actually combinations of many different fatty acids, each exerting characteristic physiological and metabolic effects. These fatty acids are generally classified as saturated, monounsaturated, or polyunsaturated. These terms refer to the number of hydrogen atoms attached to the carbon atoms of the acid chains in the fat molecule.

Saturated fatty acids in foods include palmitic and myristic acids. A common mono-unsaturated fatty acid is oleic acid, and the most common polyunsaturated fatty acid in food is linoleic acid.

Fats in foods are triglycerides combined with both saturated and unsaturated fatty acids. In general, fats containing a majority of saturated fatty acids are solid at room temperature, although some solid vegetable shortenings are up to 75 percent unsaturated. Fats containing mostly unsaturated fatty acids are usually liquid at room temperature and are called oils.

Technically, cholesterol is not a fat, but rather a fat-like substance classified as a lipid. Cholesterol is vital to life and is found in all cell membranes. It is necessary for the production of bile acids and steroid hormones.

Fats and Weight Loss

The National Cholesterol Education Program recommends dietary modification as the first treatment for elevated blood cholesterol. The recommendations are designed to reduce intake of saturated fat and cholesterol and to promote weight loss for those who are overweight.

First, limit total fat to less than 30 percent of calories, saturated fat to less than 10 percent of calories, and cholesterol to less than 300 mg. daily—similar to the U.S. Dietary Guidelines and those espoused by most health authorities today.

Research shows that even the most motivated individuals have difficulty with long-term compliance to very low-fat diets, in part because they dislike the taste of some low-fat foods. Although fat substitutes will not compensate for poor dietary habits, these ingredients may be a help to many persons trying to eat healthful, balanced diets.

Consumers have expressed a demand for foods lower in calories and fat. As more companies continue to apply their research and development skills to this challenge, a number of innovative products are sure to follow.

Moderation in fat and cholesterol consumption is only one aspect of good nutrition. Variety, moderation, and balance of all foods is the most prudent approach for the general population. Moreover, combining a well-balanced diet with getting plenty of exercise, maintaining proper weight, avoiding smoking, and controlling diseases such as hypertension and diabetes is the best approach to a healthy lifestyle.

The chief cause

for going off a diet

is trading what we want the "most"

for

what we want in the "moment."

NOTES TO MYSELF

YOUR pH BALANCE

Your acid/alkaline balance (pH) is a major factor in your health. Your energy levels, immunity, and emotional outlook are based on your pH.

Most people are not particularly interested in understanding or learning about their pH. However, if you would like to monitor your pH for the first few weeks of this diet, the information provided here will assist you in doing this.

The term pH refers to the parts of hydrogen concentration in a solution (such as blood, urine, or saliva). The scale runs from 1 to 14, with 7 being neutral. Below 7 is acid; above 7 is alkaline. The body's preference is 7.2-7.4, which is slightly alkaline. No one pH is better than another.

The body's pH has a dynamic state of ebb and flow. The body goes to great lengths to regulate the homeostasis of its preferred blood pH. However, most people's body environment could use a little assistance. An imbalance in the blood chemistry means that many of the natural functions could be inhibited.

A pH that is too acidic could contribute to rheumatoid arthritis, diabetes, lupus, tuberculosis, and some cancers. Too alkaline a pH could contribute to constipation, flu, heart trouble, indigestion, bacterial and viral infections, and some other diseases.

You can purchase the "pHydrion Lo Buff" pH paper from a holistic health professional. Measure the second urination of the day. Let urine run onto a small piece of the pH tape. Compare the color with the color chart on the tape container. It should be between 6.2 and 7.0 If it runs high or low, the information provided here will assist you in bringing your pH back into balance.

Measure the pH each day for a few weeks. You will begin to understand the different pH cycles that your body goes through. Soon you will notice when your pH is out of balance without having to use the tape. Become aware of your moods, body functions, and environment during these first few weeks of measuring.

Too yellow (acidic) - one of these may help:

Cool bath with salt and baking soda or Epsom salt

Pineapple juice 6 oz., other fruit juices except cranberry

Fresh vegetable juice

Herbal teas: chamomile, peppermint, fenugreek, red clover, hibiscus

Deep breathing

Rapid exercise

Lemon juice in water

Cold shower

Too green/blue (alkaline):

Hot bath with vinegar or mustard (1 oz. for 14 minutes in warm water)

Hot shower

Herbal teas: desert herb, spearmint, shave grass (horsetail), raspberry leaf, buchu

Low-stress proteins: soaked seeds, sprouts, sesame tahini, sauerkraut, sour pickles, olives

Brisk walk with long strides

Building proper pH (alkaline reserve and acid activity) promotes a depth of resources and stability, rather than radical swings.

Do not attempt fasting
in any form
without supervision
from your physician.

158

A WARRIOR'S MEAL

We knocked on the door, and Joseph opened it. "Come in, come in," he said enthusiastically, as if welcoming us to his home. It did, in fact, look like a home. Thick carpets covered the floor of the small waiting room. Heavy, polished, rough-hewn tables were placed around the room, and the soft straight-backed chairs looked like antiques. Tapestries hung on the walls, except for one wall almost completely hidden by a huge aquarium of colorful fish. Morning light poured through a skylight overhead. We sat directly below it, in the warm rays of the sun, occasionally shaded by clouds drifting overhead. Joseph approached us, carrying two plates over his head. With a flourish, he placed them in front of us, serving Socrates first, then me. "Ah, it looks delicious!" said Socrates, tucking his napkin into the neck of his shirt. I looked down. There before me, on a white plate, were a sliced carrot and a piece of lettuce. I stared at it in consternation. At my expression, Socrates almost fell out of his chair laughing and Joseph had to lean against a table. "Ah," I said, with a sigh of relief. "It is a joke, then." Without another word, Joseph took the plates and returned with two beautiful wooden bowls. In each bowl was a perfectly carved, miniature replica of a mountain. The mountain itself was a blended combination of cantaloupe and honeydew melon. Small chunks of walnuts and almonds, individually carved, became brown boulders. The craggy cliffs were made from apples and thin slices of cheese. The trees were made of many pieces of parsley, each pruned to a perfect shape, like bonsai trees. An icing of yogurt capped the peak. Around the base were halved grapes and a ring of fresh strawberries. I sat and stared. "Joseph, it's too beautiful. I can't eat this; I want to take a picture of it." Socrates, I noticed, had already begun eating, nibbling slowly, as was his manner. I attacked the mountain with gusto and was almost done, when Socrates suddenly started gobbling his food. I realized he was mimicking me. I did my best to take small bites, breathing deeply between bites as he did, but it seemed frustratingly slow. "The pleasure you gain from eating, Dan, is limited to the taste of the food and the feeling of a full belly. You must learn to enjoy the entire process. The hunger beforehand, the careful preparation, setting an attractive table, chewing, breathing, smelling, tasting, swallowing, and the feeling of lightness and energy after the meal. Finally, you can enjoy the full and easy elimination of the food after it's digested. When you pay attention to all these elements, you'll begin to appreciate simple meals; you won't need as much food. The irony of your present eating habits is that while you fear missing a meal, you aren't fully aware of the meals you do eat." "I'm not afraid of missing a meal," I argued. "I'm glad to hear that. It will make the coming week easier for you. This meal is the last one you'll be having for the next seven days." Soc proceeded to outline a purifying fast that I was to begin immediately. Diluted fruit juice or plain herb teas were to be my only fare. "But, Socrates, I need my protein and iron to help my leg heal; I need my energy for gymnastics." It was no use. Socrates could be a very unreasonable man. We helped Joseph with a few chores, talked for a while, thanked him, and left. I was already hungry. While we walked back toward campus, Socrates summarized the disciplines I was to follow until my body regained its natural instincts. "In a few years, there will be no need for rules. For now, however, you're to eliminate all foods that contain refined sugar, refined flour, meat, and eggs, as well as drugs including coffee, alcohol, tobacco, or any other nonuseful food. Eat only fresh, unrefined, unprocessed foods, without chemical additives. In general, make breakfast a fresh-fruit meal, perhaps with cottage cheese or yogurt. Your lunch, your main meal, should be a raw salad, baked or steamed potato, perhaps some cheese, and whole-grain bread or cooked grains. Dinner should be a raw salad and, on occasion, lightly steamed vegetables. Make good use of raw, unsalted seeds and nuts at every meal." "I guess by now you're quite an expert on nuts, Soc," I grumbled. On the way home, we passed by a neighborhood grocery store. I was about to go inside and get some cookies when I remembered that I was no longer allowed to eat store-bought cookies for the rest of my life! And for the next six days and twenty-three hours, I wouldn't be eating anything at all. "Socrates, I'm hungry." "I never said that the training of a warrior would be a piece of cake!"

— *A passage from The Way of the Peaceful Warrior, by Dan Millman*

THOUGHTS ABOUT A ONE-DAY FAST

Some feel that it is a good idea to not eat one day a month or even one day a week. This allows the body the chance to rest and cleanse itself.

Some people drink only water on their fast day. Others dedicate the day to only drinking teas and juices. Some eat only fruit. Water only is probably the best one-day fast, but not everyone can stick to that at first. You could even try every three months to start and see if it is suited to your particular lifestyle and health patterns.

Fasting is strictly a personal decision. Many people have many thoughts about whether or not fasting is beneficial. The only way to decide is to try it! You and your body will know if it is something that can provide you with additional health and well-being.

Here is some information with regard to fasting on a once-a-week basis: The idea of fasting one day a week has profound implications. In the Biblical account of creation, God rested on the seventh day. Our bodies run on seven-day cycles. For women, four seven-day cycles make up the menstrual cycle, bringing a time of cleansing and renewal. Millions of people are admonished to fast one day a week by their religions. Some donate their day's food to the homeless people of their community.

A one-day-a-week fast adds up to 52 days a year—a significant rest for the digestive system, a significant saving for the food budget, and a significant gain in health and longevity.

Those who fast one day a week say that they have a sense of living more in accord with the body's natural cycles. There seems to be always a special sense of being for those who live in accord with nature. Such a practice eliminates the need for prolonged therapeutic fasts unless a person wishes to fast at length for some special reason.

Should you want to participate in the one-day fast, it's recommended that you allow yourself a full 24-hour period, which means you have your supper one evening, begin fasting as you awaken the next morning, fast all day, and do not break your fast until the following morning. Drink pure water throughout your fast. In the natural life rhythms, Friday is the optimal fast day, but from a nutritional health perspective any day will do.

People who fast one day a week usually notice a balancing trend in their health—weight normalizes, allergies clear up, constipation is relieved, and the immune system strengthens.

'By my body teach the mind.
'Tis the mind that makes the body rich.'
— Shakespeare

CHAPTER NINE

Time Out

ACKNOWLEDGING YOURSELF

When was the last time you treated yourself to something you really loved? Many people don't know how to nurture themselves—especially without using food as the reward. This exercise will support you in identifying and appreciating the good things about yourself. Fill this form in at the beginning of each week.

After the eight weeks, go back and see if you can feel where or if you became comfortable or more comfortable with the ways that you nurture yourself now and the way you may have changed your lifestyle to accommodate yourself and your needs. How have you allowed others to be a part of this process for you? Has this changed in eight weeks or has it stayed the same?

'Whether in life or in a diet,
only you
can deprive yourself!'

HEART TIME

Place your focus of attention into the region of your heart for a moment and take a deep breath.

The heart is a very precious organ in the body. Without the heart, there is no beating of life in the physical organism. Without the heart there is no juice in the system, nothing to keep it going here, alive and functioning, moving as a unit. So the heart, then, is by far the most essential ingredient of the body. The heart is the element around which everything else functions.

The heart is more powerful, more potent, and has more wisdom than anything else in the physical organism. That is not to say that it is better, it is simply the essential item needed for being alive in the physical arena.

So, your heart will become the focus of your attention in this exercise. Every day, take five minutes to focus in on the area in your heart. Five minutes, at least, every day. You can make this part of any other quiet time or personal nurturing time that you have set aside for yourself. But it is a time where you will spend five minutes of focused energy in the area of your heart.

In your heart lies the seed of your spirit. And within your spirit lies the current of your soul. Again, without the heart there is no key to that unit called your body. And when you travel in this area you will begin to understand your inner self. This is an understanding that will take place without words, without thoughts, without analysis. It is an understanding between you and your spirit, which is a knowing more than anything else. You are going to learn about your know-ingness. And you are going to do this simply by being in this place where you are in your center with your self.

That place is in your heart.

So let us experiment right now. Allow yourself to close your eyes and take a deep breath and move gently into the area where your heart is. Moving gently. It's so simple. And when you feel yourself in that place where that is the only thing that is important to you at this time, you may rest. You may rest in there. And perhaps you might feel as if you would like to take a nap in there. But you will not fall asleep.

You will be relaxed but you will remain alert. Alert to your senses. This is a natural part of your senses. It is deeper, more profound, and larger than any state within the realm of your mental mind. That is why this is a place without words, without analysis.

It is a state of being still, where you are totally the receiver. Like the receiver on a battery, you begin to receive input from yourself. That is all there is to do right now—receive input from yourself.

Take note of what you are feeling. What do you feel in here, in your heart? What is it like? Hold your focus. Stay focused and alert to your feelings. Simply be a receiver. Open to all the information that is available and coming to you at this time from your inner self. Focus yourself on your feeling of your sense.

This is a sensory experience. For most of you, holding your focus is a challenge. Holding your focus in this way, without input from your mind, is the challenge that faces you. Always return your focus to your heart as often as you feel yourself slipping away from it. Gently come back to focus in your heart.

Record and write down what it is that you sense and feel in those moments with your heart. This will be very, very important information for you. And never analyze it. Simply keep it as it is when it comes to you. Write it down without any evaluation or judgment. Just as it is. Plain and simple.

—*by R.T.*

A SPECIAL EXERCISE

This is an exercise of a different sort. Most of you, by now, are well aware of the body exercises, especially the ones that go along with most diets. However, the following is a very special kind of exercise designed especially for you. This exercise is created to assist you in the ability to come closer to your inner self. The focus with diets is usually on the outer self. However, the outer you is often a visual manifestation of the you inside.

This exercise is a way to help you establish a loving and nurturing closeness with your innermost personal self, to begin to see what you really see from the inside out.

There is a lot of emphasis on nurturing in this section. Most of you are probably experts on nurturing others, but when it comes to taking care of *your* needs and your own nurturing, you don't rate high on the list.

Please take the time to read the list on the following pages. Read the questions through several times until you really get a feeling for them.

Relax and close your eyes. Slowly count down from twenty-five. Once you reach zero, begin to ask yourself any of the questions that you remember. You don't have to remember them in order, and you don't have to remember all of them. You also don't need to open your eyes to refer to the list. Only ask yourself those questions that you remember.

This is not a test! This is merely an exercise to begin moving you into yourself. A quiet time. A time to be still. A time to be with yourself. Once you have asked a question, stay quiet and listen. After a few minutes, begin to move your energy (thoughts) from your head area down into the area of your heart. Let go of any thoughts at this point. Just be still . . . and listen.

Make an effort to do this exercise once in the morning and once in the evening. It should take only a few minutes. Read over the questions a few times before you begin your exercise. Eventually, ask each of these questions during your exercise. Take your time. After a while you may enjoy extending the time and asking your own questions.

BEING STILL

1. Am I relaxed?

2. Am I fully present in the moment?

3. In what ways do I compromise myself? My body?

4. Would I rather be doing something else? What? Why?

5. How do I feel about being still?

6. Does my mind chatter try to control my efforts to be still?

7. Do I love *all* of me?

8. Am I willing to hear the truth about the questions I ask myself?

9. Am I resisting this exercise?

10. Am I listening to my heart-talk?

11. Do I feel connected to myself?

12. Do I let my thoughts just pass through and not disturb me?

13. What messages am I receiving from my body?

14. Am I angry? Where in my body do I keep my anger?

15. Do I feel safe?

16. Am I letting go of my thoughts?

17. What am I holding on to? Where in my body do I hold?

18. What judgments do I have about this?

19. Am I detached from the answers?

20. Am I worried about something? Why?

21. Do I feel silly?

22. What does it feel like at the source of myself?

23. Where is my center?

24. Do I feel nurtured? By whom? By myself?

25. How does it feel to do something for myself?

26. Am I feeling light?

27. Do I feel guilty?

28. Do I feel that I'm not good enough?

29. Do I feel heavy?

30. Am I feeling scattered?

31. Do I feel that I'm moving deeper into myself?

32. Am I conscious?

33. Where is my energy?

34. How is this exercise affecting my body?

35. Do I feel resentments? Toward myself or toward others?

36. Is this exciting?

37. Am I focused on what I'm doing?

38. How does it feel to be all by myself? Inside myself?

39. Does my anger make me powerless? Why?

40. Do I feel fat? Where? How does my fat feel?

41. Am I breathing? Do I feel my breath within my body?

42. What am I afraid of?

43.   Am I listening?

44.   Am I comfortable about nurturing myself?

45.   Is this effortless?

46.   Where in my body do I keep my fear?

47.   Where do I hold my pain? My hurts?

48.   What am I feeling?

49.   What part of me holds my happiness?

50.   Have I quieted my mind-talk?

51.   Do I feel at peace with myself and my body?

52.   What does intimacy mean to me?

53.   How does my "inner child" feel?

54.   Am I looking forward to doing this again?

*"Can you imagine what it might feel like
to not have any cares or worries?
Merely to be quiet, calm, and at peace all the time?"*

The Ten Scrolls

1. Today I begin a new life, I will form good habits. My vigor will increase, my enthusiasm will rise, my desire to meet the world will overcome every fear I once knew at sunrise. Today I begin a new life.

2. I will greet this day with love in my heart. From this moment I have not time to hate, only time to love. I will greet this day with love, and I will succeed.

3. I will persist until I succeed. Each obstacle I will consider as a mere detour to my goal and a challenge to my profession. I will forget the happenings of the day that is gone, and greet the new sun with confidence that this will be the best day of my life. I will persist. I will win.

4. I am nature's greatest miracle. I have unlimited potential. Nature knows not defeat. I will win, for I am unique. I am nature's greatest miracle.

5. I will live this day as if it were my last. I will waste not a moment mourning yesterday's defeats; yesterday is buried forever. Each hour of this day I will cherish. Each minute of today will be more fruitful than hours of yesterday. My last must be my best. I will live this day as if it were my last; and if it is not, I will give thanks.

6. Today I will be master of my emotions. Weak is he who permits his thoughts to control his actions; strong is he who forces his actions to control his thoughts. I am prepared to control whatever personality awakes in me each day. I will become master of myself. I will become great.

7. I will laugh at the world. No creature can laugh except man. I will enjoy today's happiness today. I will laugh at my failures and they will vanish in clouds of new dreams. I will be happy. I will be successful.

8. Today I will multiply my value a hundredfold. I will set goals for today, the week, the month, the year, and my life. Today I will surpass every action which I performed yesterday. I will never be content with my performance. Today I will multiply my value a hundredfold.

9. My dreams are worthless, my plans are dust, my goals are impossible. All are of no value unless they are followed by action. I will act now. My procrastination which has held me back was born of fear, and I now recognize this secret mined from the depths of all courageous hearts. Now I know that to conquer fear I must always act without hesitation and the flutters in my heart will vanish. Now I know that action reduces the lion of terror to an ant of equanimity. I will act now. I will act now. I will act now. I will repeat these words again and again and again each day until the words become as much a habit as my breathing. When I awake I will say them and leap from my cot while the failure sleeps yet another hour. Now is all I have. Tomorrow is reserved for the lazy. I will act now. Success will not wait. This is the time. This is the place. I am the person. I will act now.

10. I will pray for guidance.

Oh Creator of all things, help me. For this day I go out into the world naked and alone, and without your hand to guide me I will wander far from the path which leads to success and happiness.

Spare me sufficient days to reach my goals; yet help me to live this day as though it be my last.

Guide me. Help me. Show me the way.

Let me become all you planned for me when my seed was planted and selected by you to sprout in the vineyard of the world. Guide me, God.

—*Og Mandino*

HOW TO LOVE YOURSELF

by Louise L. Hay

1. **STOP ALL CRITICISM.** Criticism never changes a thing. Refuse to criticize yourself. Accept yourself exactly as you are. Everybody changes. When you criticize yourself, your changes are negative. When you approve of yourself, your changes are positive.

2. **DON'T SCARE YOURSELF.** Stop terrorizing yourself with your thoughts. It's a dreadful way to live. Find a mental image that gives you pleasure (mine is yellow roses), and immediately switch your scary thought to a pleasure thought.

3. **BE GENTLE AND KIND AND PATIENT.** Be gentle with yourself. Be kind to yourself. Be patient with yourself as you learn the new ways of thinking. Treat yourself as you would someone you really loved.

4. **BE KIND TO YOUR MIND.** Self-hatred is only hating your own thoughts. Don't hate yourself for having the thoughts. Gently change your thoughts.

5. **PRAISE YOURSELF.** Criticism breaks down the inner spirit. Praise builds it up. Praise yourself as much as you can. Tell yourself how well you are doing with every little thing.

6. **SUPPORT YOURSELF.** Find ways to support yourself. Reach out to friends and allow them to help you. It is being strong to ask for help when you need it.

7. **BE LOVING TO YOUR NEGATIVES.** Acknowledge that you created them to fulfill a need. Now you are finding new, positive ways to fulfill those needs. So lovingly release the old negative patterns.

8. **TAKE CARE OF YOUR BODY.** Learn about nutrition. What kind of fuel does your body need to have optimum energy and vitality? Learn about exercise. What kind of exercise can you enjoy? Cherish and revere the temple you live in.

9. **MIRROR WORK.** Look into your eyes often. Express this growing sense of love you have for yourself. Forgive yourself looking into the mirror. Talk to your parents looking into the mirror. Forgive them too. At least once a day say "I love you, I really love you!"

10. **DO IT NOW!** Don't wait until you get well, or lose the weight, or get the new job, or the new relationship. Begin now—do the best you can!

'Every minute of the day
you are choosing
what the next minute will bring.'

FIRST WEEK

PERSONAL ACHIEVEMENTS THIS WEEK:_____

_____

GOOD QUALITIES I ACKNOWLEDGE:_____

_____

WHAT I LIKE ABOUT MY BODY:_____

_____

HOW DO I ACCENTUATE MY GOOD FEATURES?_____

_____

NONFOOD REWARDS THAT I LOVE:_____

_____

WHAT DO I AGREE TO DO TO NURTURE MYSELF THIS WEEK?

_____

HOW DOES IT FEEL TO NURTURE MYSELF?_____

_____

HAVE I ALLOWED OTHERS TO NURTURE ME?_____ HOW?_____

_____

SECOND WEEK

PERSONAL ACHIEVEMENTS THIS WEEK:_____

_____

GOOD QUALITIES I ACKNOWLEDGE:_____

_____

WHAT I LIKE ABOUT MY BODY:_____

_____

HOW DO I ACCENTUATE MY GOOD FEATURES?_____

_____

NONFOOD REWARDS THAT I LOVE:_____

_____

WHAT DO I AGREE TO DO TO NURTURE MYSELF THIS WEEK?

_____

HOW DOES IT FEEL TO NURTURE MYSELF?_____

_____

HAVE I ALLOWED OTHERS TO NURTURE ME?_____HOW?

_____

THIRD WEEK

PERSONAL ACHIEVEMENTS THIS WEEK:_____

_____

GOOD QUALITIES I ACKNOWLEDGE:_____

_____

WHAT I LIKE ABOUT MY BODY:_____

_____

HOW DO I ACCENTUATE MY GOOD FEATURES?_____

_____

NONFOOD REWARDS THAT I LOVE:_____

_____

WHAT DO I AGREE TO DO TO NURTURE MYSELF THIS WEEK?

_____

HOW DOES IT FEEL TO NURTURE MYSELF?_____

_____

HAVE I ALLOWED OTHERS TO NURTURE ME?_____HOW?

_____

FOURTH WEEK

PERSONAL ACHIEVEMENTS THIS WEEK:_____

_____

GOOD QUALITIES I ACKNOWLEDGE:_____

_____

WHAT I LIKE ABOUT MY BODY:_____

_____

HOW DO I ACCENTUATE MY GOOD FEATURES?_____

_____

NONFOOD REWARDS THAT I LOVE:_____

_____

WHAT DO I AGREE TO DO TO NURTURE MYSELF THIS WEEK?

_____

HOW DOES IT FEEL TO NURTURE MYSELF?_____

_____

HAVE I ALLOWED OTHERS TO NURTURE ME?_____HOW?

_____

FIFTH WEEK

PERSONAL ACHIEVEMENTS THIS WEEK:_____

_____

GOOD QUALITIES I ACKNOWLEDGE:_____

_____

WHAT I LIKE ABOUT MY BODY:_____

_____

HOW DO I ACCENTUATE MY GOOD FEATURES?_____

_____

NONFOOD REWARDS THAT I LOVE:_____

_____

WHAT DO I AGREE TO DO TO NURTURE MYSELF THIS WEEK?

_____

HOW DOES IT FEEL TO NURTURE MYSELF?_____

_____

HAVE I ALLOWED OTHERS TO NURTURE ME?_____HOW?

_____

SIXTH WEEK

PERSONAL ACHIEVEMENTS THIS WEEK:_____

_____

GOOD QUALITIES I ACKNOWLEDGE:_____

_____

WHAT I LIKE ABOUT MY BODY:_____

_____

HOW DO I ACCENTUATE MY FEATURES?_____

_____

NONFOOD REWARDS THAT I LOVE:_____

_____

WHAT DO I AGREE TO DO TO NURTURE MYSELF THIS WEEK?

_____

HOW DOES IT FEEL TO NURTURE MYSELF?_____

_____

HAVE I ALLOWED OTHERS TO NURTURE ME?_____HOW?

_____

SEVENTH WEEK

PERSONAL ACHIEVEMENTS THIS WEEK:_____

_____

GOOD QUALITIES I ACKNOWLEDGE:_____

_____

WHAT I LIKE ABOUT MY BODY:_____

_____

HOW DO I ACCENTUATE MY GOOD FEATURES?_____

_____

NONFOOD REWARDS THAT I LOVE:_____

_____

WHAT DO I AGREE TO DO TO NURTURE MYSELF THIS WEEK?

_____

HOW DOES IT FEEL TO NURTURE MYSELF?_____

_____

HAVE I ALLOWED OTHERS TO NURTURE ME?_____HOW?

_____

EIGHTH WEEK

PERSONAL ACHIEVEMENTS THIS WEEK:_____

_____

GOOD QUALITIES I ACKNOWLEDGE:_____

_____

WHAT I LIKE ABOUT MY BODY:_____

_____

HOW DO I ACCENTUATE MY GOOD FEATURES?_____

_____

NONFOOD REWARDS THAT I LOVE:_____

_____

WHAT DO I AGREE TO DO TO NURTURE MYSELF THIS WEEK?

_____

HOW DOES IT FEEL TO NURTURE MYSELF?_____

_____

HAVE I ALLOWED OTHERS TO NURTURE ME?_____HOW?

_____

CHAPTER TEN

Out House

SUGGESTED READING LIST

A Course in Miracles
—Foundation for Inner Peace

Betrayal • The Evolution of Self-Shaping
–Sandra Parent   www.ebookstand.com

Born to Win
—Muriel James

Breaking Free from Compulsive Eating,
Feeding the Hungry Heart, and *Why Weight?*
—Geneen Roth

Co-Dependence
—Anne Wilson Schaef

Codependent No More and *Beyond Co-Dependency*
—Melody Beattie

Creative Visualization, Living in the Light,
and *Return to the Garden*
—Shakti Gawain

Energy & Additions, The Liver Triad, and *The Pro-Vita Diet*
—Jack Tipps, N.D., Ph.D., and A. Stuart Wheelwright
(ordered through Insight Press, 4001 Manchaca Road,
Austin, TX 78704)

Diets Don't Work
—Bob Schwartz

Fat Is a Family Affair
—Judi Holis, Ph.D.

Fat Is a Feminist Issue
—Susie Orbach

Getting Unstuck: Breaking Through the Barriers to Change
—Sidney B. Simon

How to Be Your Own Best Friend
—Mildred Newman

How to Get Rid of Fat
—Charles L. Pelton

I'm Okay, You're Okay
—Thomas A. Harris, M.D.

Keeping It Off
—Robert H. Colvin and Susan C. Olson

Mary Ellen's Help Yourself Diet Plan
—Mary Ellen Pinkham

The Mists of Avalon
—Marion Zimmer Bradley

Road Less Traveled
—M. Scott Peck

Stress, Sanity and Survival: How to Stop Making Impossible Demands On Yourself
—Robert Woolfolk and Frank Richardson

T-Factor Diet
—Martin Katahn, Ph.D.

Talking with Nature
—Michael J. Roades

Take It Off and Keep It Off
—Roger C. Katz and D. Balfour Jeffrey

The Book of Hope: How Women Can Overcome Depression
—Helen DeRosis and Victoria Pellegrino

"The New Diet Mindset"
—Psychology Today, June 1989

The Only Diet There Is
—Sondra Ray

The Quickening, The Force, Miracles, Affirmations, Life Was Never Meant to Be a Struggle, and *Whispering Winds of Change, Weight Loss for the Mind*   —Stuart Wilde   www.whitedoveinternational.com

184

The Thin Connection
—Martin M. Schiff, M.D.

The Transparent Self
—Sidney M. Jourard

The Twelve Steps for Everyone
— CompCare Publishers, 1977

The Yo-Yo Syndrome Diet
—Doreen L. Virtue

Understanding—Eliminating Stress and Finding Serenity in Life and Relationships
—Jane Nelson, Ed.D.

When I Say No, I Feel Guilty
—Manuel Smith

Why Am I Afraid to Tell You Who I Am?
—John Powell

Women Who Run With the Wolves
—Clarissa Pinkola Estes, Ph.D.

You Can Heal Your Life and Heal Your Life
—Louise Hay (books and tapes: Hay House, Los Angeles, CA)

AUDIO PROGRAMS:

Energy Anatomy
-Caroline Myss, Ph.D.

Your Personality, Your Health, and Your Life
–Carol Ritberger, Ph.D.

THINGS I WANT TO REMEMBER

Some points of my philosophy:

We are each 100% responsible for all of our experiences.

Every thought we think is creating our future.

The point of power is always in the present moment.

Everyone suffers from self-hatred and guilt.

The bottom line for everyone is, "I'm not good enough."

It's only a thought, and a thought can be changed.

Resentment, criticism and guilt are the most damaging patterns.

When we really love ourselves, everything in our life works.

We must release the past and forgive everyone.

We must be willing to begin to learn to love ourselves.

Self-approval and self-acceptance in the now

are the key to positive changes.

—From You Can Heal Your Life by Louise Hay

THE BUTTERFLY

I remembered one morning when I discovered a cocoon in the bark of a tree, just as a butterfly was making a hole in its case and preparing to come out. I waited awhile, but it was too long appearing and I was impatient. I bent over it and breathed on it to warm it. I warmed it as quickly as I could and the miracle began to happen before my eyes, faster than life.

The case opened, the butterfly started slowly crawling out and I shall never forget my horror when I saw how its wings were folded and crumpled; the wretched butterfly tried with its whole trembling body to unfold them. Bending over it, I tried to help it with my breath. In vain.

It needed to be hatched out patiently. And the unfolding of the wings should be a gradual process in the sun. Now it was too late. My breath had forced the butterfly to appear all crumpled, before its time. It struggled desperately and, a few seconds later, died in the palm of my hand.

That little body is, I do believe, the greatest weight I have on my conscience. For I realize today that it is a mortal sin to violate the great laws of nature.

We should not hurry, we should not be impatient, but we should confidently obey the eternal rhythm.

—From Zorba the Greek by Nikos Kazantzakis

In the quietness of my heart,
the deep valleys of my mind,
and the very being of my soul . . .
I am what I am
and that will always be love!

WEIGH OUT STORIES

Like most women my age, I've read enough books on diets to get a Ph.D. Your book is by far the absolute best! Especially for women! We need to understand and encourage the entire wellness of our beings - so we can help lead the way to heal ourselves, our families, and our planet. Healing begins with the self. —Sherry Bolling

This has to be the best weight loss and maintenance program I have ever participated in. It incorporates all of the essential elements necessary to confidently lose weight in a safe and controlled environment. I highly recommend it to my family and friends all the time. I totally agree with the opinion that you must change your lifestyle to keep the weight off on a permanent basis. This book gives the answers to long overdue questions. I don't think there is any one answer to the overweight problems that most women face, but I do believe that this program brings together the safety of traditional medicine along with the alternatives of holistic ideas. I'm full of energy and a new sense of accomplishment. If I can do this after so many false attempts, I can do anything. —Rose Aubrey

I lost over thirty pounds and my life has changed for the better. Friends, family and my husband are so proud of the way I look and feel. Having lost three dress sizes made shopping much easier and it's great to be able to wear fun, fashionable clothes again. The maintenance program has helped me keep the weight off and continue my life being the "new me!" — Vikki Berndt

I am among the group of people that have tried everything to lose weight. I have used powders, packets, and fad pills. The Grapefruit diet, Popcorn diet, Hollywood diet, bar bells, machines, packaged foods, frozen foods, fasting, creams, saran wraps, and even tried to steam it off. Finally my physicians told me about this program and I figured "why not" I've tried everything else. Two months later I had lost more pounds than I had lost altogether with all the other stuff combined. This diet really works! I had several of my friends ask me how I did it and I tell them about this program. Now that I've lost the weight I still continue to stop in once a month to see Kathy the nurse. She tells me how terrific I look and I tell her its because of her and her support. —Nick Rose

"Whatever you can do,
or dream you can do, begin it.
Boldness has genius, power and magic in it.
Begin it NOW !" — *Goethe*

NOTES TO MYSELF

*'I accept myself the way I am
and the way I am not.'*